Starving the Anxiety Gremlin

FOR CHILDREN AGED 5–9

by the same author

Starving the Anger Gremlin for Children Aged 5–9
A Cognitive Behavioural Therapy Workbook
on Anger Management
ISBN 978 1 84905 493 5
eISBN 978 0 85700 885 5

Starving the Anger Gremlin
A Cognitive Behavioural Therapy Workbook
on Anger Management for Young People
ISBN 978 1 84905 286 3
eISBN 978 0 85700 621 9

Starving the Anxiety Gremlin
A Cognitive Behavioural Therapy Workbook
on Anxiety Management for Young People
ISBN 978 1 84905 341 9
eISBN 978 0 85700 673 8

Starving the Stress Gremlin
A Cognitive Behavioural Therapy Workbook
on Stress Management for Young People
ISBN 978 1 84905 340 2
eISBN 978 0 85700 672 1

Banish Your Body Image Thief
A Cognitive Behavioural Therapy Workbook on
Building Positive Body Image for Young People
ISBN 978 1 84905 463 8
eISBN 978 0 85700 842 8

Banish Your Self-Esteem Thief
A Cognitive Behavioural Therapy Workbook on
Building Positive Self-Esteem for Young People
ISBN 978 1 84905 462 1
eISBN 978 0 85700 841 1

of related interest

The Panicosaurus
Managing Anxiety in Children Including
Those with Asperger Syndrome
K.I. Al-Ghani
Illustrated by Haitham Al-Ghani
ISBN 978 1 84905 356 3
eISBN 978 0 85700 706 3

Frog's Breathtaking Speech
How Children (and Frogs) Can Use Yoga
Breathing to Deal with Anxiety, Anger and Tension
Michael Chissick
Illustrated by Sarah Peacock
ISBN 978 1 84819 091 7
eISBN 978 0 85701 074 2

Starving the Anxiety Gremlin

FOR CHILDREN AGED 5–9

A COGNITIVE BEHAVIOURAL THERAPY
WORKBOOK ON ANXIETY MANAGEMENT

KATE COLLINS-DONNELLY

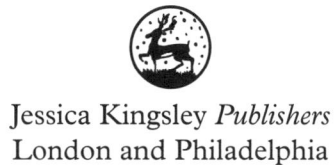

Jessica Kingsley *Publishers*
London and Philadelphia

First published in 2014
by Jessica Kingsley Publishers
73 Collier Street
London N1 9BE, UK
and
400 Market Street, Suite 400
Philadelphia, PA 19106, USA

www.jkp.com

Copyright © Kate Collins-Donnelly 2014
Anxiety Gremlin illustrations copyright © Tina Gothard 2014

All rights reserved. No part of this publication may be reproduced in any material form (including photocopying of any pages other than those marked with a ✓, or storing it in any medium by electronic means and whether or not transiently or incidentally to some other use of this publication) without the written permission of the copyright owner except in accordance with the provisions of the Copyright, Designs and Patents Act 1988 or under the terms of a licence issued by the Copyright Licensing Agency Ltd, Saffron House, 6–10 Kirby Street, London EC1N 8TS. Applications for the copyright owner's written permission to reproduce any part of this publication should be addressed to the publisher.

All pages marked ✓ may be photocopied for personal use with this programme, but may not be reproduced for any other purposes without the permission of the publisher.

Warning: The doing of an unauthorised act in relation to a copyright work may result in both a civil claim for damages and criminal prosecution.

Library of Congress Cataloging in Publication Data
Collins-Donnelly, Kate.
  Starving the anxiety gremlin for children aged 5-9 : a cognitive behavioural therapy workbook on anxiety management / Kate Collins-Donnelly.
    pages cm
  Includes bibliographical references.
  ISBN 978-1-84905-492-8 (alk. paper)
  1. Anger--Juvenile literature. 2. Anger in children--Juvenile literature.
  3. Cognitive therapy for children--Juvenile literature. I. Title.
  BF723.A4C655 2014
  618.92'85220651--dc23
                          2014006413

British Library Cataloguing in Publication Data
A CIP catalogue record for this book is available from the British Library

ISBN 978 1 84905 492 8
eISBN 978 0 85700 902 9

Printed and bound in Great Britain by Bell and Bain Ltd, Glasgow

The authorized representative in the EEA is Hachette Ireland,
8 Castlecourt Centre, Dublin 15, D15 XTP3, Ireland (email: info@hbgi.ie)

Contents

ACKNOWLEDGEMENTS 7

ABOUT THE AUTHOR 8

1. Why Read This Book? 9
2. Let's Meet a Mystery Creature! 19
3. Let's Learn about Feelings! 29
4. What Is Anxiety? 41
5. Things We Get Anxious About 59
6. Why We Get Anxious 71
7. Our Anxious Bodies 89
8. Our Anxious Behaviours 103
9. The Effects Anxiety Can Have 117
10. Starving the Anxiety Gremlin Strategies 129
11. Your Anxiety Dos and Don'ts! 161

12. **Completing Your Mission to Starve the Anxiety Gremlin!** **165**

    ACTIVITY, PUZZLE AND QUIZ ANSWERS 179

    INFORMATION FOR PARENTS AND PROFESSIONALS 189

    REFERENCES 192

Acknowledgements

First, I would like to thank Maria for her motivation, inspiration, support and guidance. I would also like to thank all the children, parents, practitioners and colleagues who have inspired me to develop this workbook. Further thanks go to everyone whom I have worked with at Jessica Kingsley Publishers, especially my editor Caroline, for their invaluable help with all my books to date. It is always a joy to work with you. Thank you also to Tina Gothard for her brilliant Anxiety Gremlin illustrations used throughout this workbook. Tina, it was a pleasure to work with you.

About the Author

Hi! I'm Kate, and I have worked for several years providing support for children, young people and their parents on the emotional issues that children and young people face today, including anxiety. I have also provided training and guidance for professionals from a variety of disciplines on how to support children, young people and their families when a child or young person is suffering with issues such as anxiety. Through this work, it became evident that there was a need for a book aimed directly at children aged 5–9 years on how to manage their anxiety, and as a result, *Starving the Anxiety Gremlin for Children Aged 5–9* was born.

This book contains stories, puzzles and activities to help you learn about what anxiety is, why we get anxious, how we think, feel and act when we get anxious and the effects that anxiety can have. It also provides a step-by-step guide to managing your anxiety by starving your Anxiety Gremlin!

I hope you find this workbook fun as well as packed with useful ways to get your anxiety under control once and for all!

Happy reading and good luck with starving your Anxiety Gremlin!

Kate

1

Why Read This Book?

This book is here to help you if...

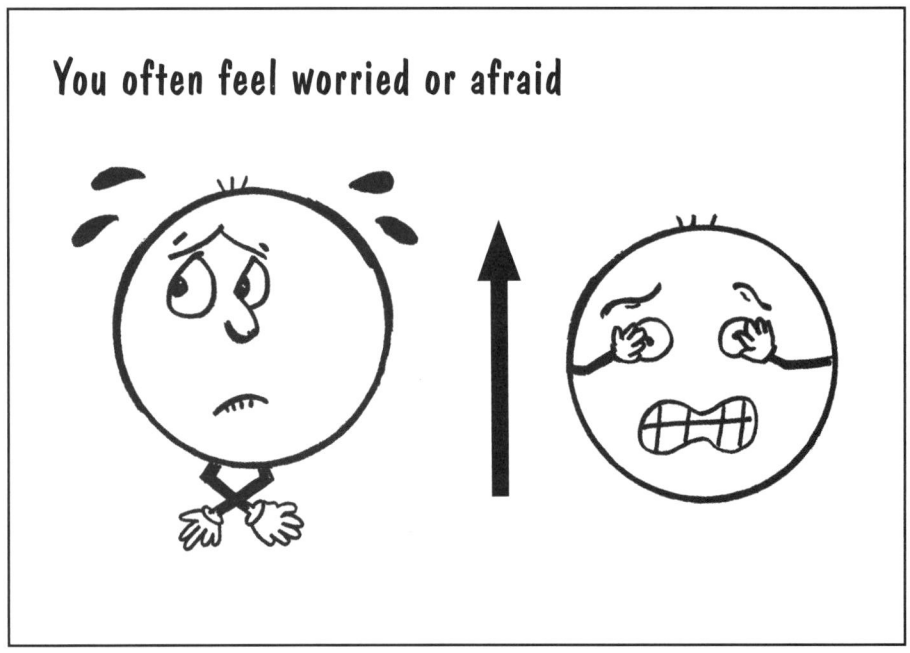

You often feel worried or afraid

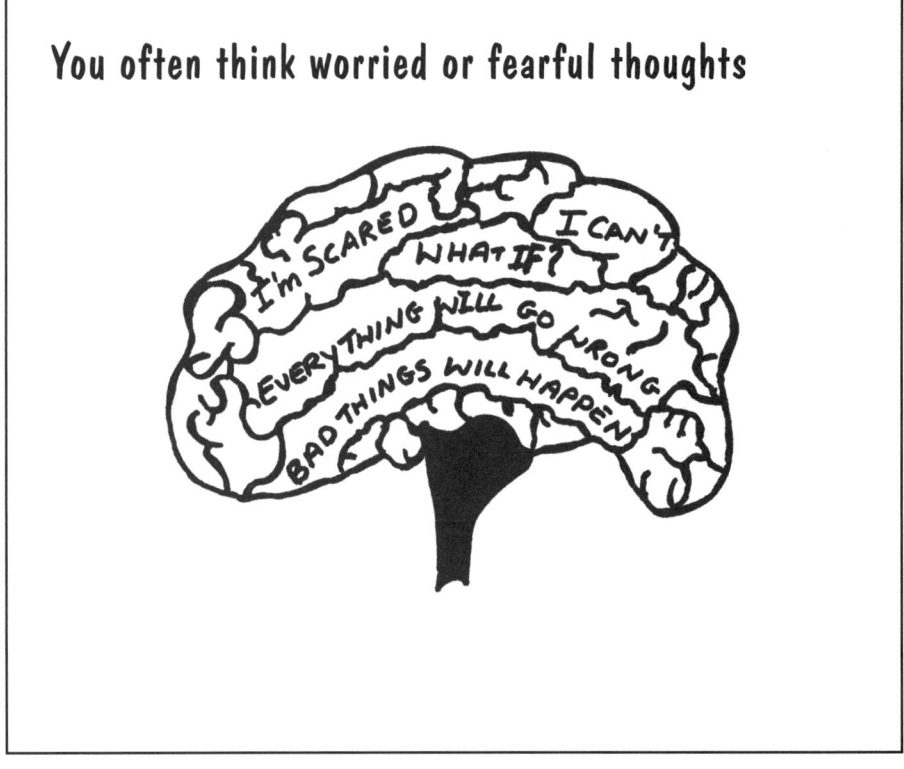

You often think worried or fearful thoughts

You avoid...

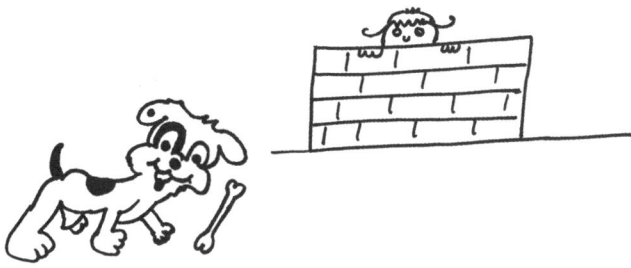

...hide...

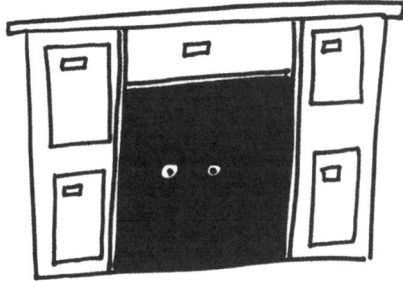

...or escape

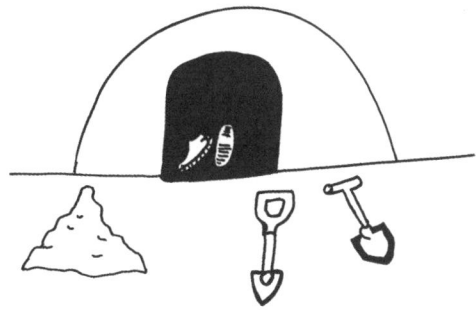

...from people, places or situations because of your worries and fears

You don't want to be apart from your parents because of your worries or fears

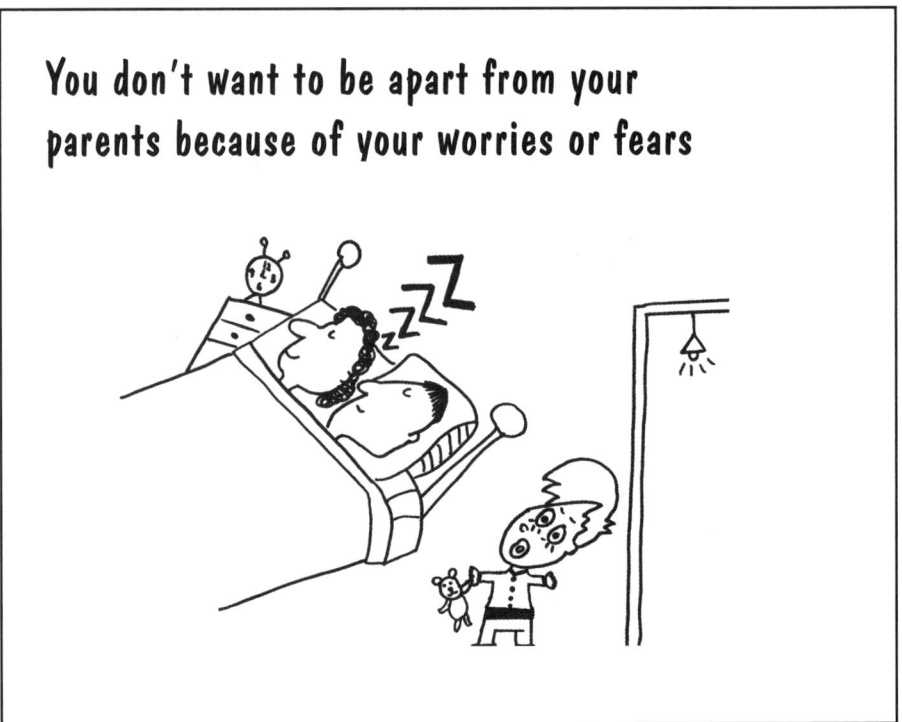

You don't want to leave your house because of your worries or fears

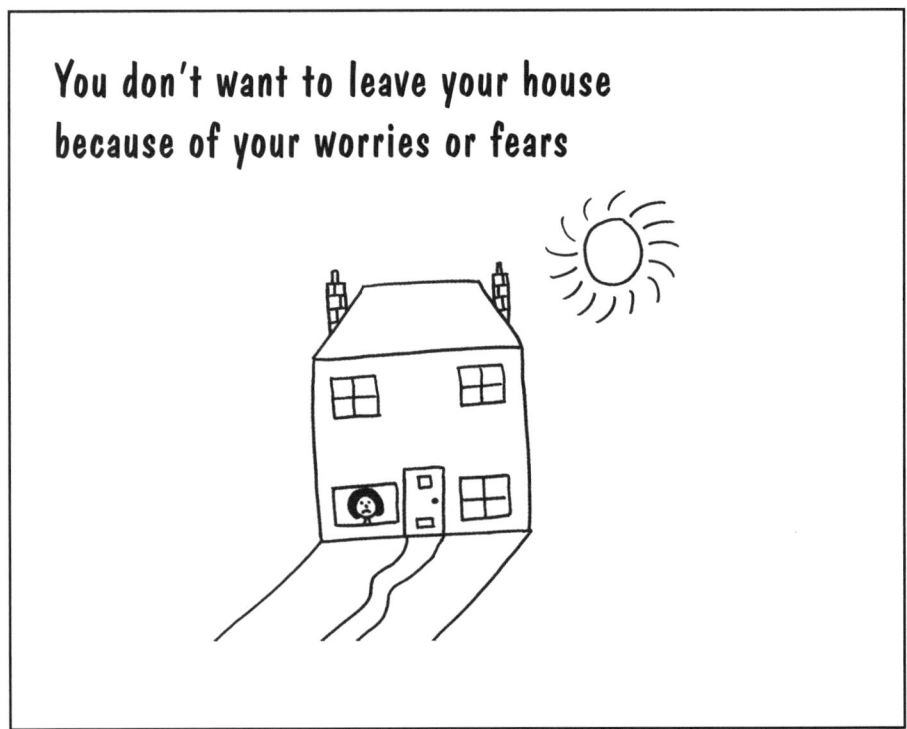

You think you need to keep saying certain words or asking people certain things to avoid bad things happening

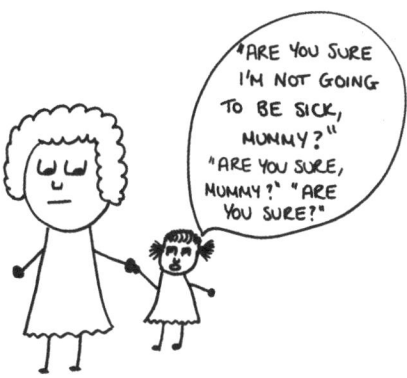

You think you need to keep washing, checking, organising, tidying, counting, touching or collecting things to avoid bad things happening

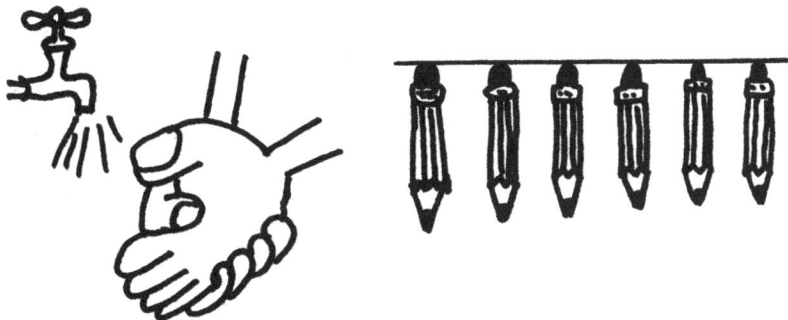

Your worries and fears make you feel bad physically

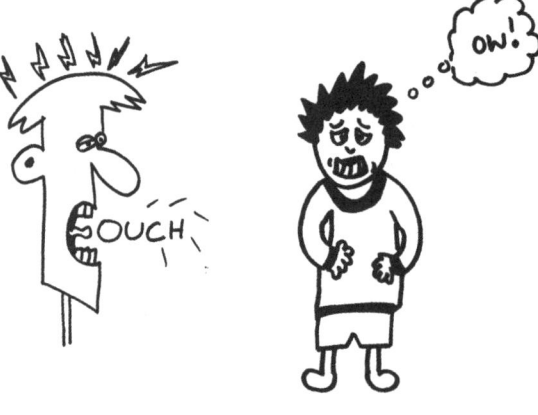

Your worries and fears are having bad effects on your life, such as missing out on doing fun or important things

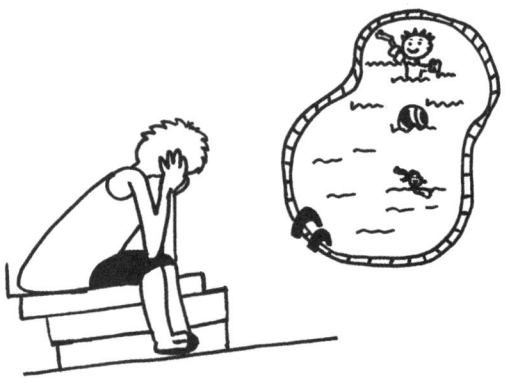

By reading this book you will learn about your own worries and fears. You will also meet a creature called the Anxiety Gremlin. The Anxiety Gremlin's favourite foods are your worries and fears. He wants you to feed him lots and lots of worries and fears so he can get bigger and bigger. But this workbook will teach you how to starve him of his favourite foods so you will...

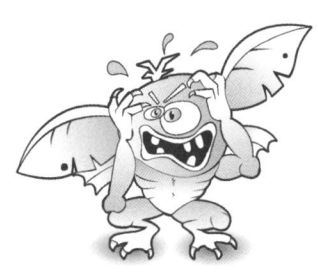

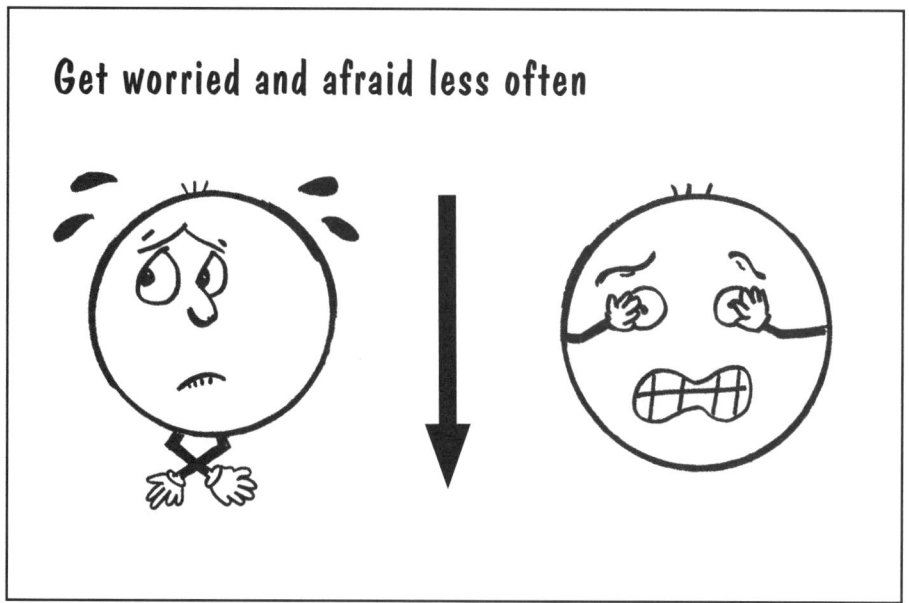

So starving your Anxiety Gremlin is your mission! And you will learn how to do this through fun puzzles, activities and stories! The answers to these puzzles and activities are at the back of the book. Plus, don't forget you can get an adult to help you along the way if you get stuck with any of them. You'll also get to draw lots of things too! And you can colour in any of the pictures you see throughout this workbook. In fact, why not colour in the pictures on the pages that you have just read?

Happy colouring!

I have one more thing to tell you about this book, which is that every time you complete a chapter you will earn two...

...rewards!

Let's take a look at what these rewards are!

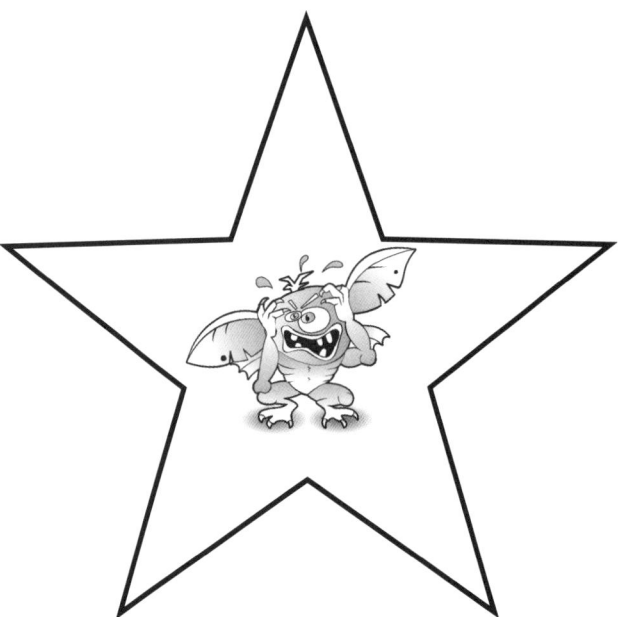

Reward 1:
The Starving the Anxiety Gremlin Star!

At the end of each chapter, you will collect a star. You can have fun colouring the stars in using whatever colours and funky patterns you like! When you have collected all 11 stars, you will have successfully completed this workbook and you will know exactly how to achieve your mission to starve your Anxiety Gremlin!

Why not colour this one in as a practice?

Reward 2:
The Just for Fun Puzzles!

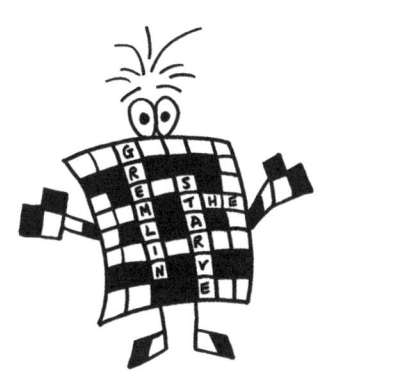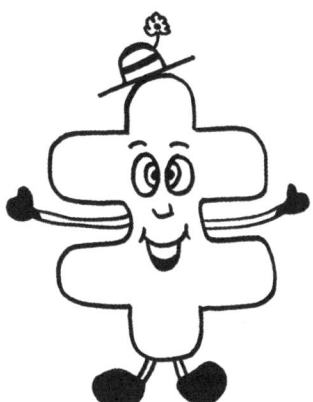

You will also have two **Just for Fun Puzzles** to choose from at the end of each chapter as a reward for all your hard work along the way. And if you like you can even complete both puzzles!

Here's a **Just for Fun Puzzle** for you to try out now!

Escape the Anxiety Gremlin!

Quick! Quick! Escape from the Anxiety Gremlin by finding the quickest way through the maze. Be careful as there are two routes out, but one will take you longer than the other!

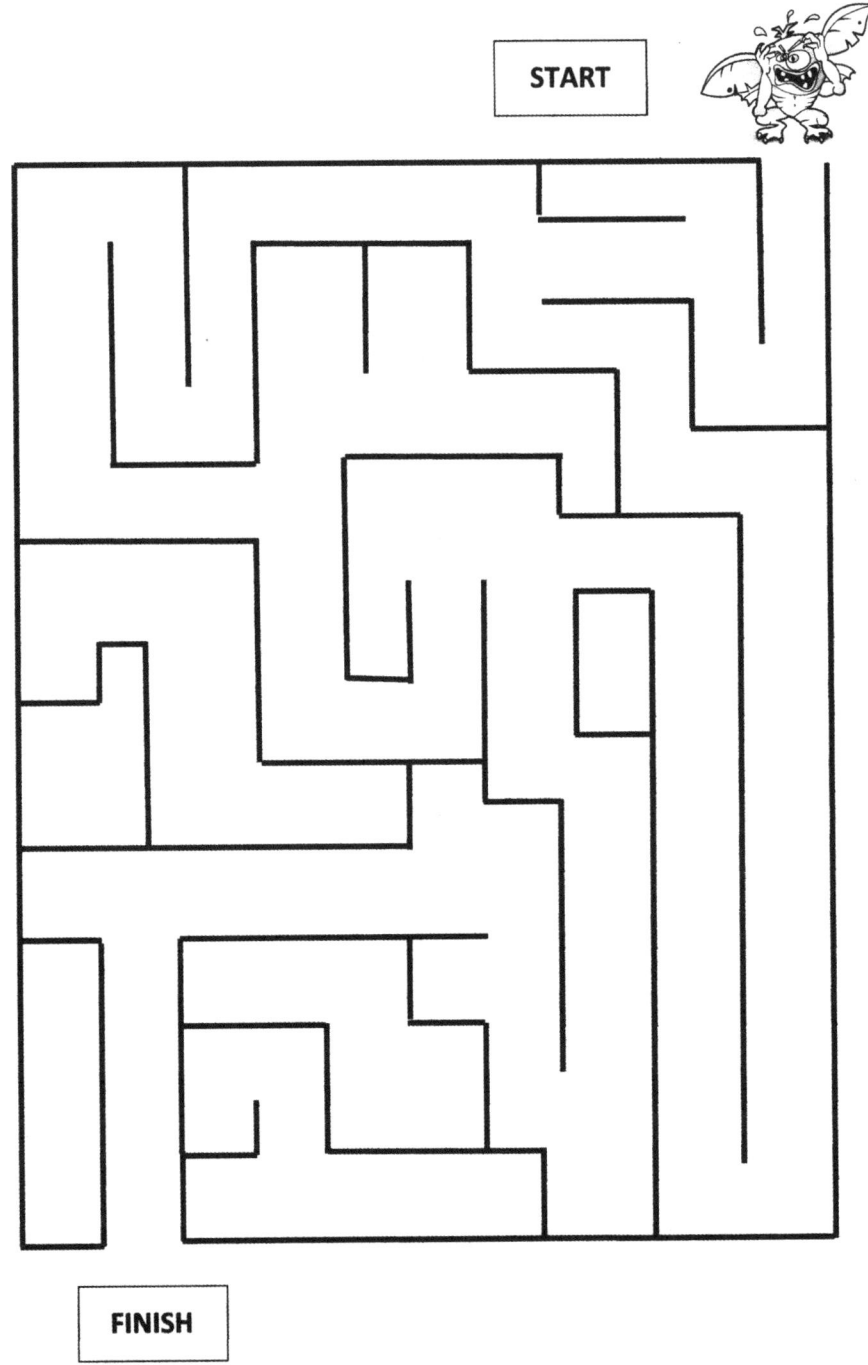

2
Let's Meet a Mystery Creature!

We're All Going on a Jungle Holiday!

You are an adventurous explorer trekking through the heart of the African jungle.

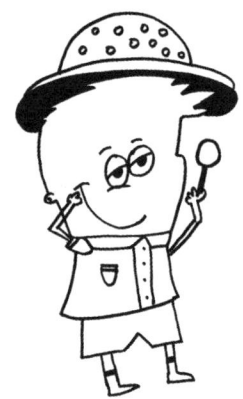

Along the way you pass lions, giraffes, monkeys, hippos, rhinos, elephants, zebras, snakes and birds of many colours. You stop to admire these amazing animals, but none of them are the mystery creature that you are looking for.

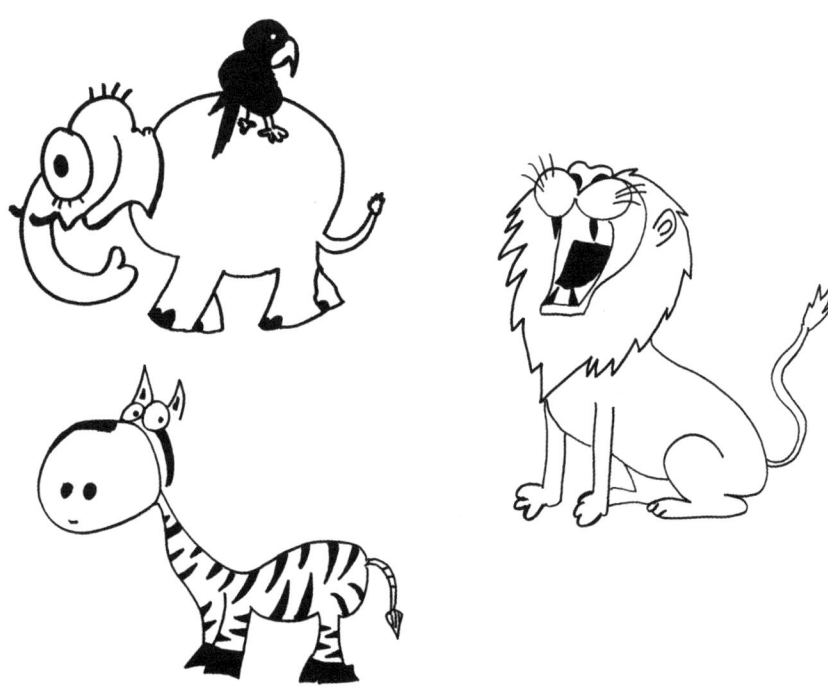

Let's Meet a Mystery Creature!

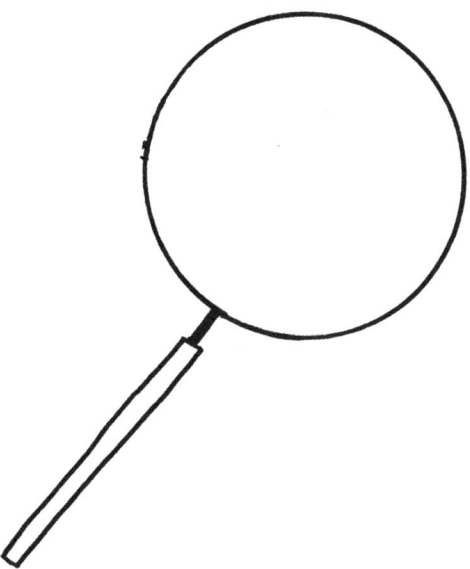

Over the page is a jungle path. As you trek along this path, you will find a number of clues to the name of the mystery creature that you seek. Follow the clues and see if you can work out who they are describing. And keep your eyes peeled as you might spot the mystery creature hidden amongst the other animals! Draw the mystery creature or write down his name in the magnifying glass at the end of the jungle trail. Also, why not colour in the animals that you pass as you move from clue to clue!

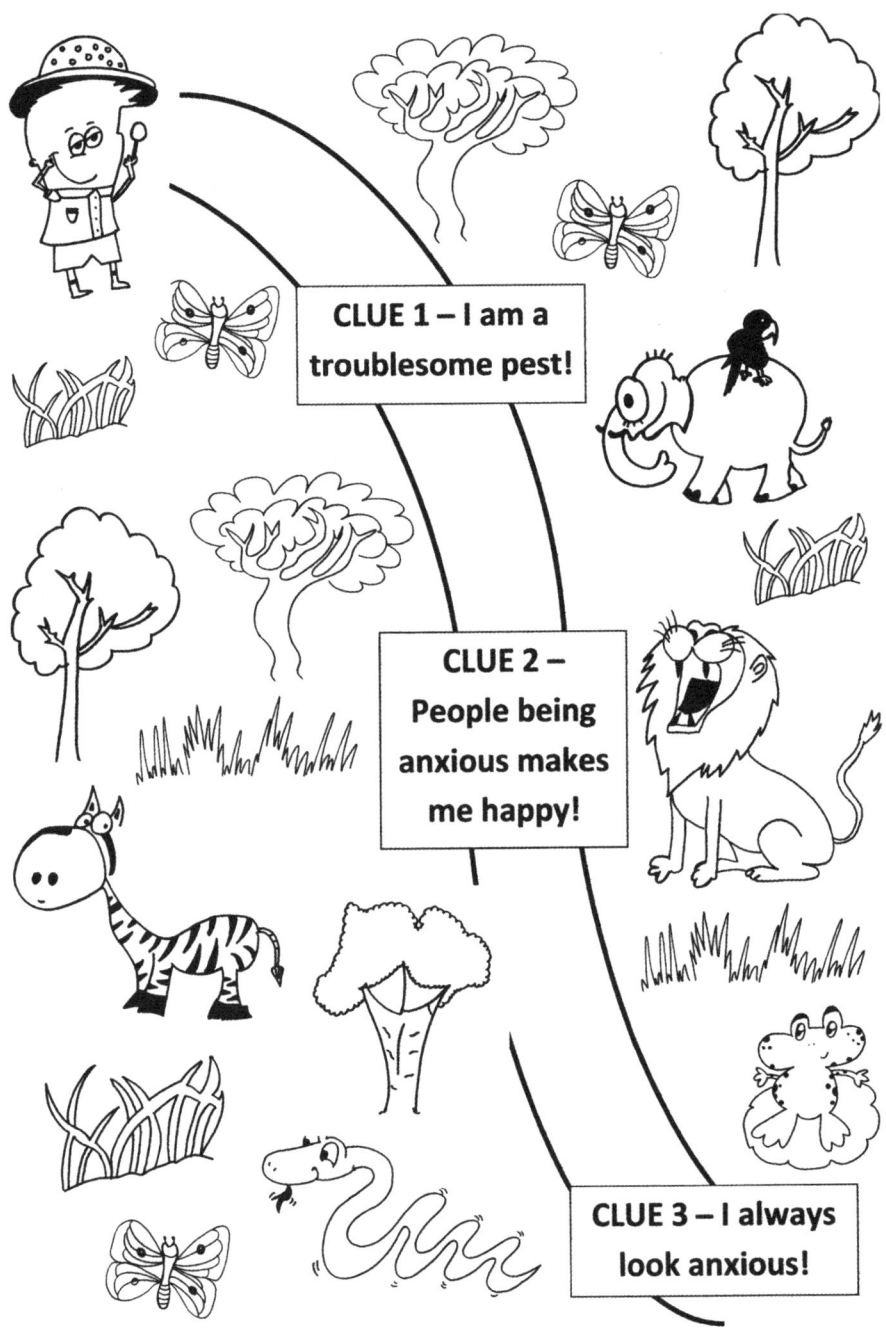

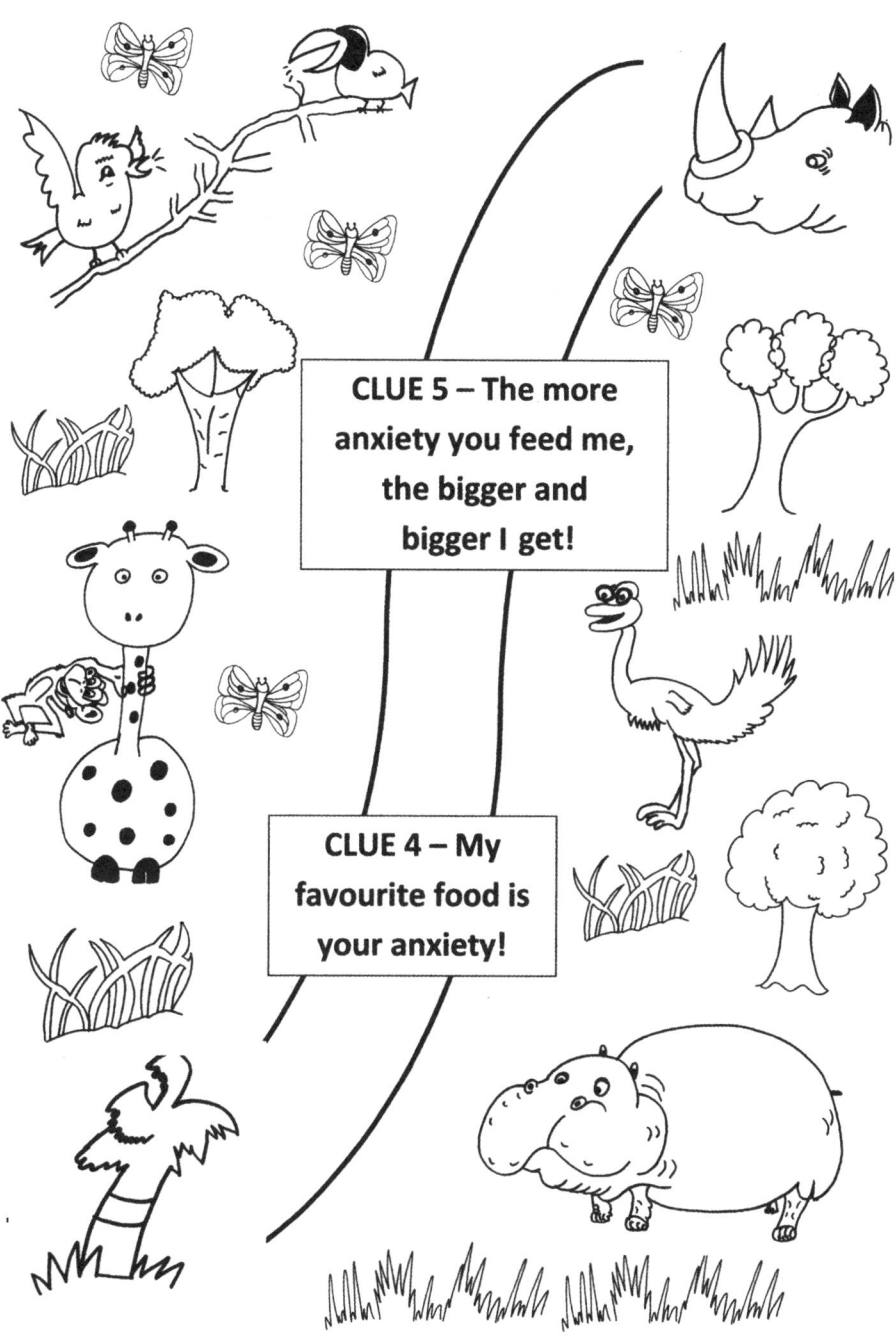

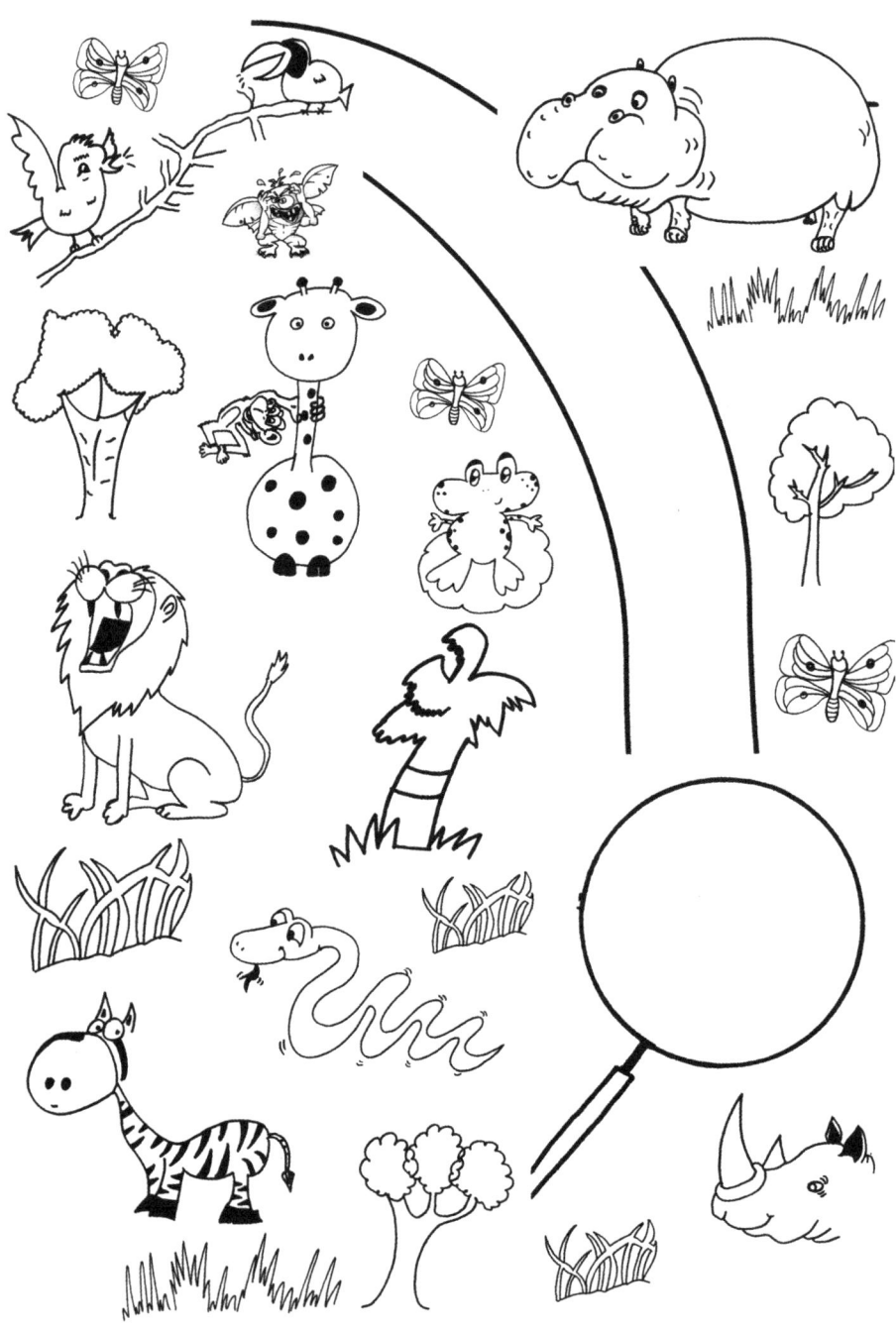

Let's Meet a Mystery Creature!   25

Here's the creature you were looking for and his name is...

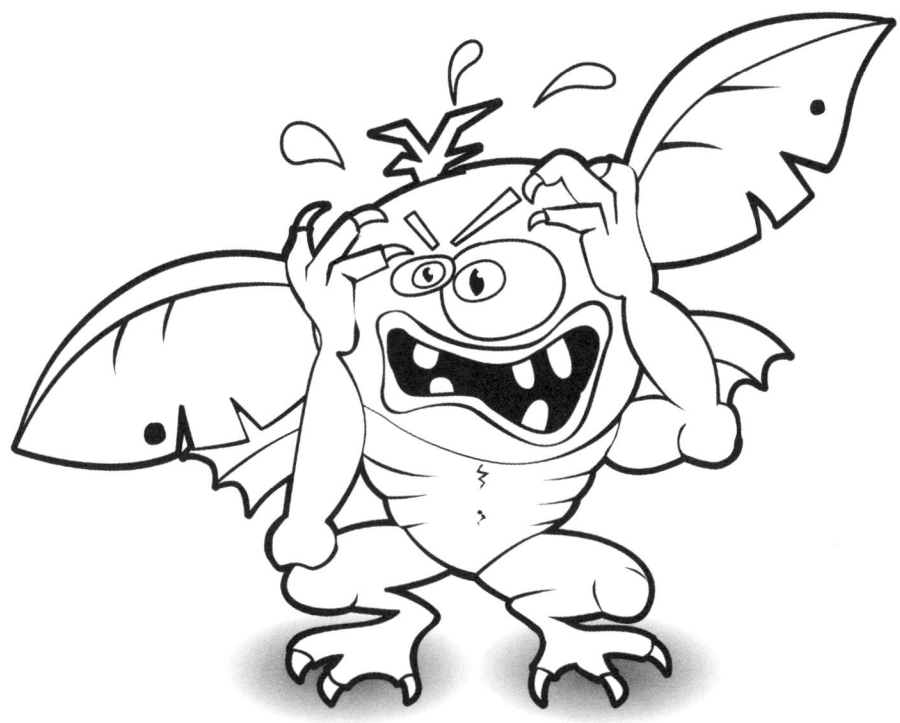

the Anxiety Gremlin!

Step 1 in starving the Anxiety Gremlin is learning who he is. You will learn more about the Anxiety Gremlin as you work through this book. But for now, why not colour him in? You can make his colours match those on the front of this book or you can choose your own – the choice is yours!

Because you have been such an amazing jungle explorer and completed Step 1 of your mission to starve your Anxiety Gremlin, you have earned your first **Starving the Anxiety Gremlin Star**! Be proud and colour in your star!

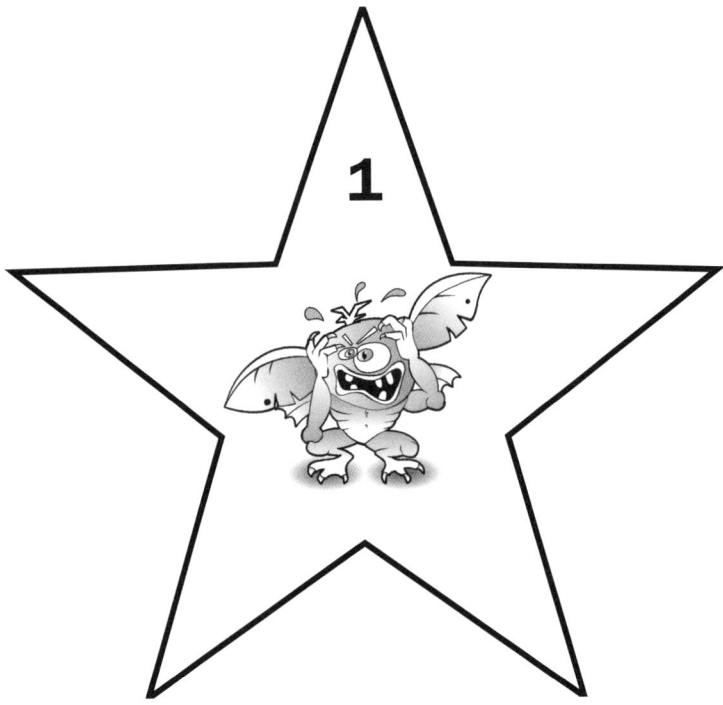

Now have a go at one or both of these **Just for Fun Puzzles** as another reward for your great work so far! Enjoy!

Gremlins Galore!

The hexagon below is full of Anxiety Gremlins and stars. How many Anxiety Gremlins are there? Write the answer on the line below.

There are _____ Anxiety Gremlins in the hexagon.

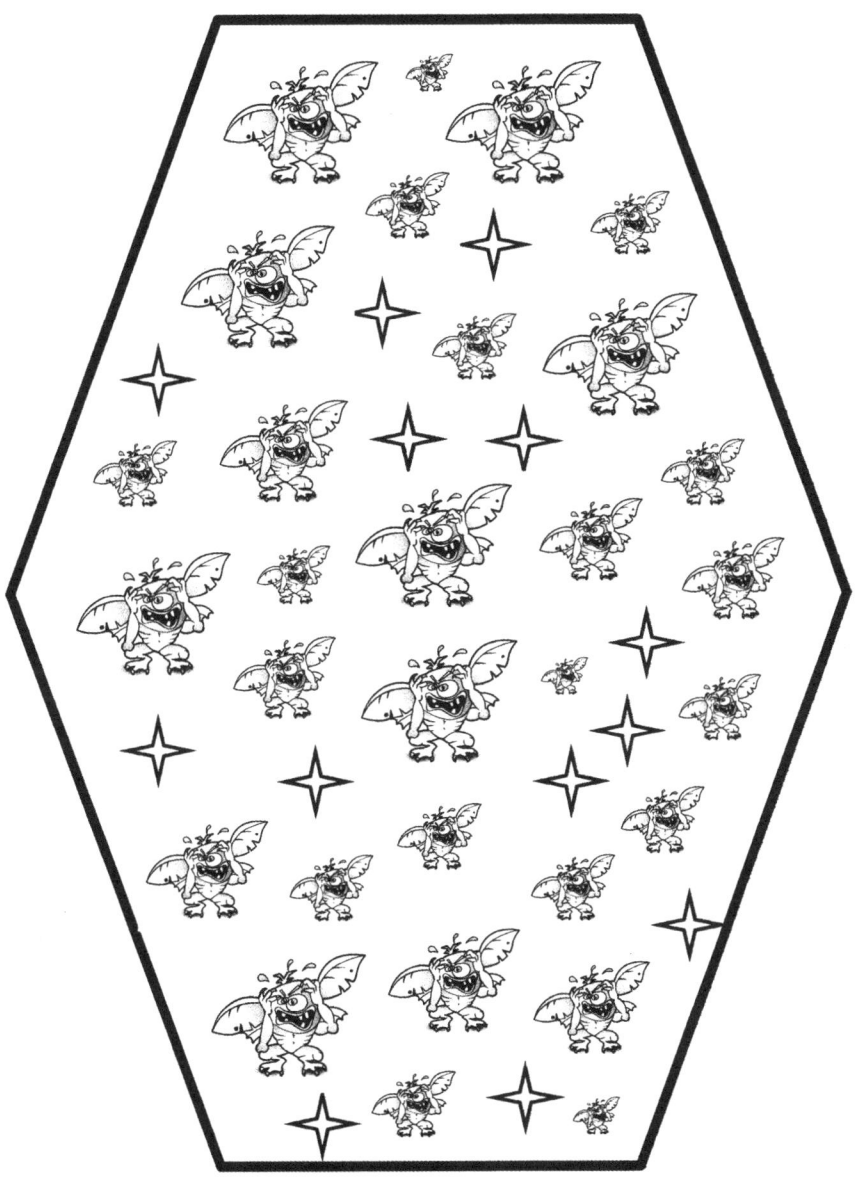

Word Multiplication!

See how many words you can make out of the letters that are used to spell...

the Anxiety Gremlin.

Write your answers in the box below. I've found two for you to start you off!

Germ

Green

3
Let's Learn about Feelings!

Learning about feelings is Step 2 in your mission to starve your Anxiety Gremlin!

Feelings, Feelings and More Feelings!

It is normal for everyone to have lots of different feelings every day, such as feeling excited about a school trip or feeling happy when you win a board game! Another word for feelings is…

emotions.

Complete the two activities below to learn about some different types of feelings.

Feelings or Not Feelings? You Decide!

Below is a picture of a girl. Your first task is to colour her in. So have fun colouring!

While you were colouring in the girl, did you notice that there are lots of words written all around her? Some of them are feelings and some aren't. Your next task is to colour in those that are feelings. Good luck!

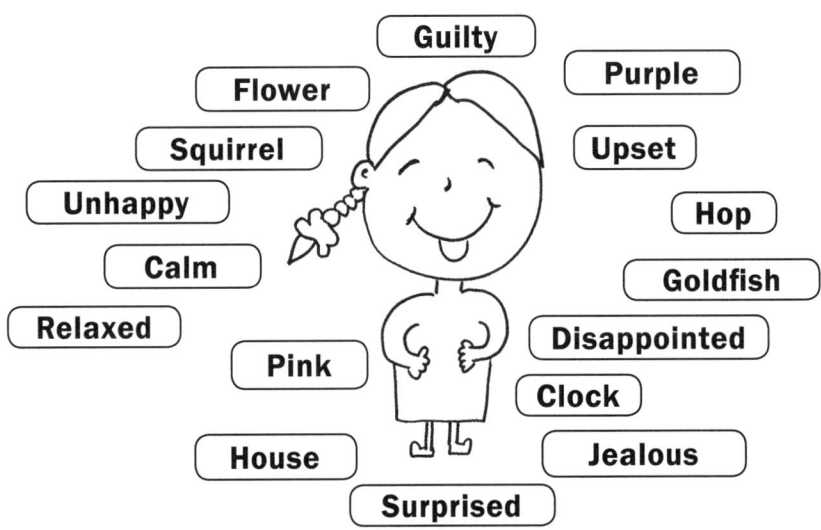

Find the Feelings!

See if you can find the following six feelings in the word search below. Circle or highlight the feelings when you find them. I've found one for you to get you started!

HAPPY   SAD   ANGRY   EXCITED   BORED   PROUD

A	T	S	A	D	H	E
N	K	B	C	M	X	X
G	V	O	Z	H	P	C
R	P	R	O	U	D	I
Y	R	E	G	K	T	T
K	J	D	Y	E	G	E
D	H	A	P	P	Y	D

Well done! You've now learnt the names of some feelings. Next let's think about how people's faces look when they have certain feelings by doing the activity below.

The Face and Feeling Mix-Up!

Below you will find six faces showing six different feelings. Each face also has a label under it with the name of a feeling. However, the naughty Anxiety Gremlin has mixed up the labels on all the faces!

See if you can work out which face should go with which label. Draw lines to match up the correct faces and feelings. Again, I've done one for you to start you off! Why not colour in the faces too for an extra bit of fun?

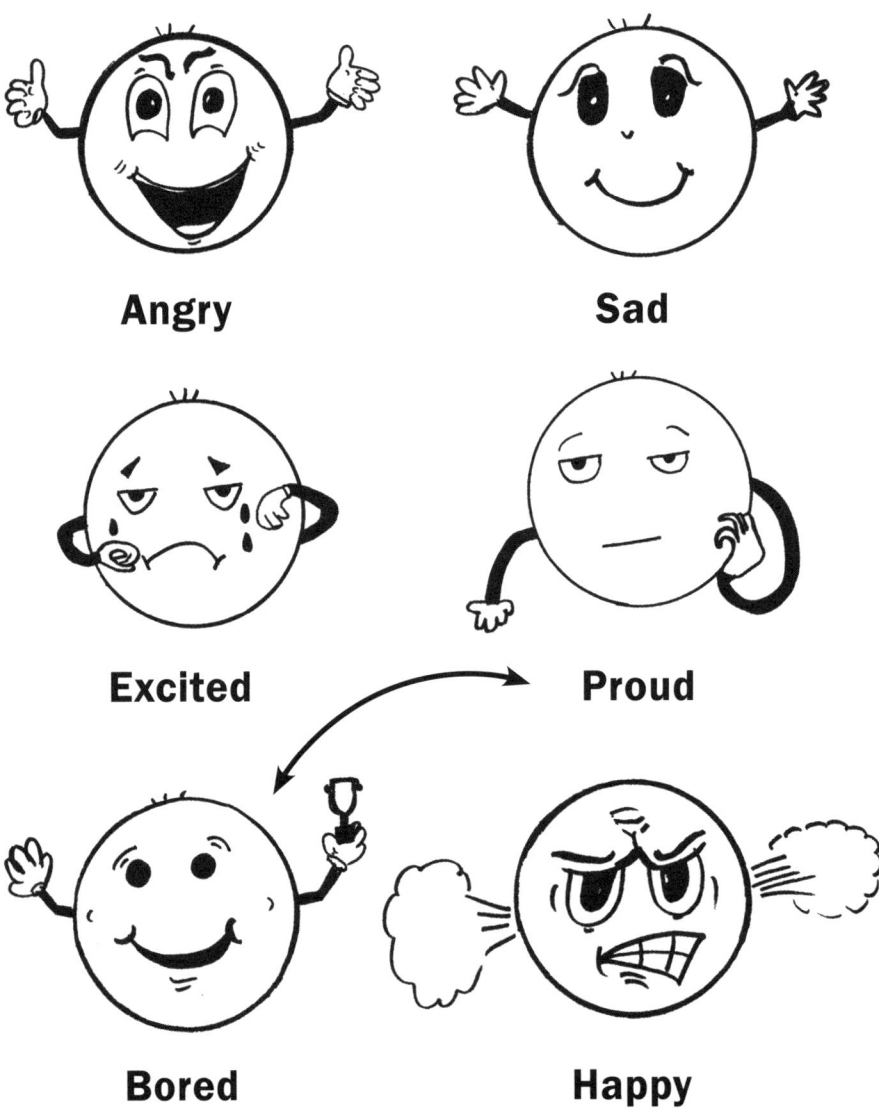

All Feelings Are Different

- You might experience some feelings **more often** than others.
- Some feelings will hang around for **a long time** but others will **come and go quickly**.
- Some feelings will be **really strong** and others will be **less strong**.

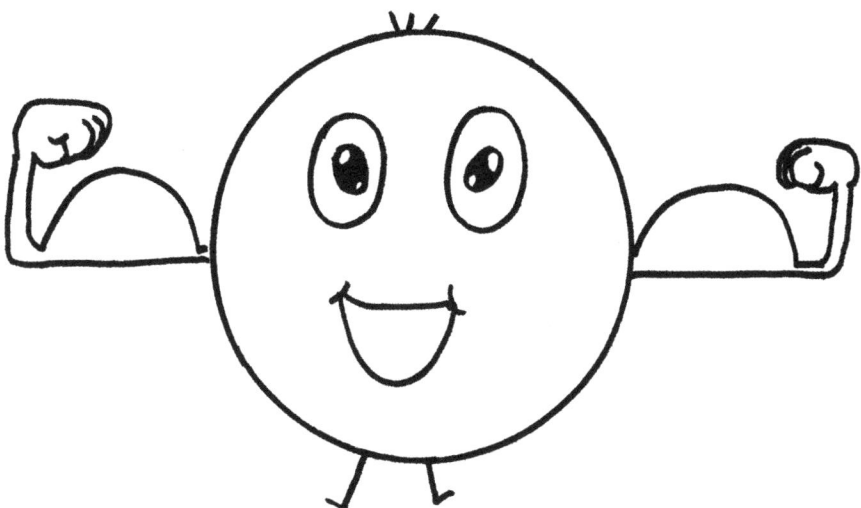

All of this is normal!

Why Do We Have Feelings?

When we have feelings, we usually have them in response to certain situations, events, places, people or objects. Below are six boxes. Each box contains a feeling. I would like you to draw a picture in each box of what makes you happy, sad, angry, excited, bored and proud.

I feel happy when...

I feel sad when...

I feel angry when…

I feel excited when…

I feel bored when...

I feel proud when...

Let's Learn about Feelings! 37

Wow! You've completed Step 2 in starving your Anxiety Gremlin by learning about feelings. Well done! Give yourself a big clap, feel proud and colour in your second **Starving the Anxiety Gremlin Star**!

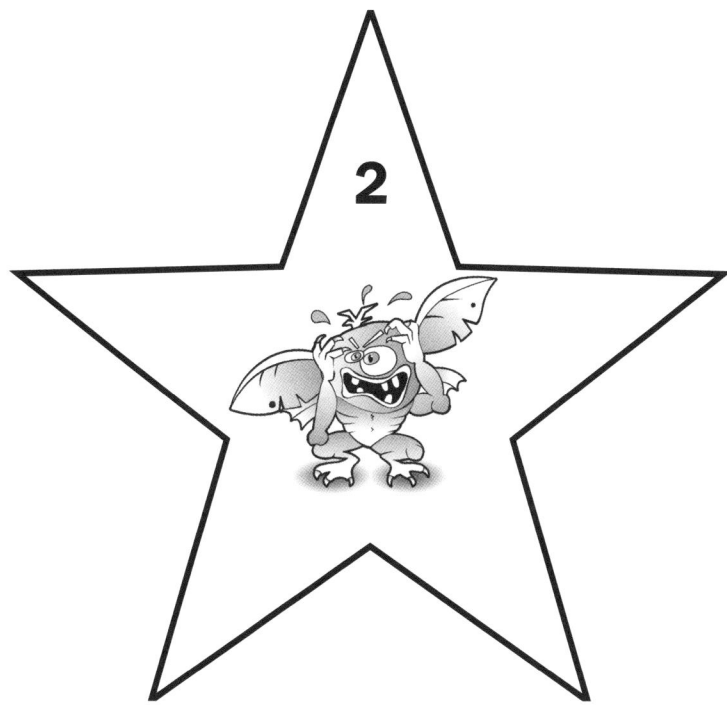

Now try completing one or both of the following **Just for Fun Puzzles** as a reward for your brilliant work so far! Have fun!

Give the Anxiety Gremlin a Makeover!

Colour in the Anxiety Gremlin using the colour code below:

1 = Blue   **2 = Red**   **3 = Green**   **4 = Orange**

Then for any parts of the Anxiety Gremlin that don't contain a number, pick your own colours. Use your imagination! Happy colouring!

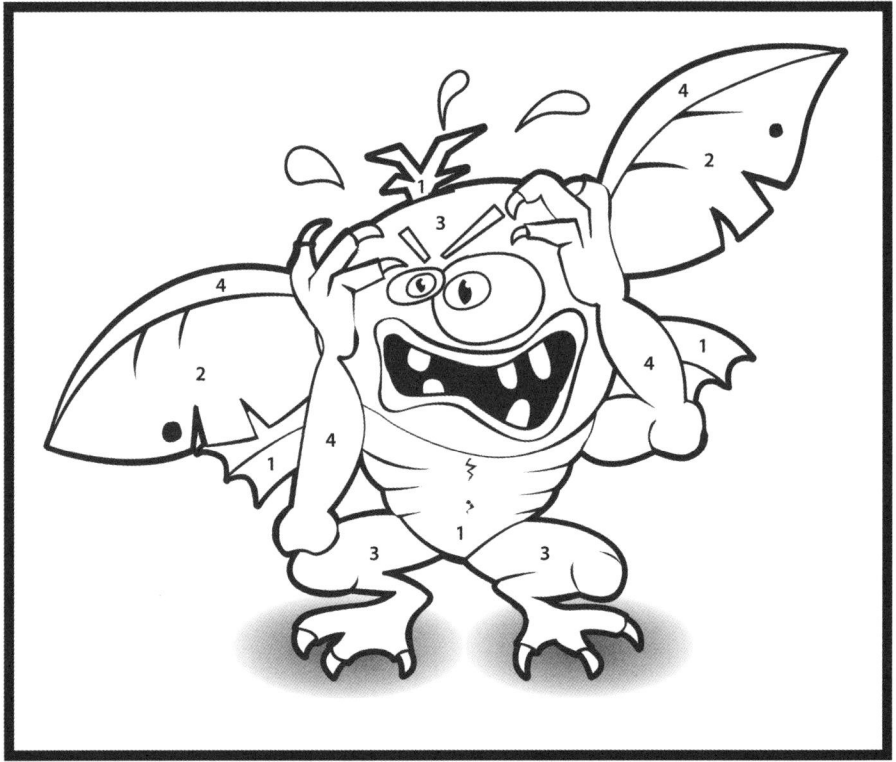

'What Am I?' Riddle

The answer to each line of the following riddle is a letter of the alphabet. When you put all these letters together in order you will spell a word. See if you can work out the word. I have given you the answer to the first and last lines of the riddle to show you how it's done. Happy solving!

My first is in FURY but never in PROUDLY [F]

My second is in RELAXED and also in UPSET [ ]

My third is in BRAVE and also in CHILLED [ ]

My fourth is in LOVE but never in ENVIOUS [ ]

My fifth is in AFRAID but never in FEARED [ ]

My sixth is in TENSE and also in DOWN [ ]

My seventh is in GIDDY and also in GLUM [ ]

My eighth is in NERVOUS and also in SAD [S]

WHAT AM I?

THE ANSWER IS F _ _ _ _ _ _ S

4
What Is Anxiety?

Step 3 in your mission to starve your Anxiety Gremlin is to learn what anxiety is.

The Anxious Feelings Spiral

Anxiety is a name that is often given to a group of three feelings. The letters in the boxes below spell out these three feelings in a spiral shape. Can you spot all three? Colour in each word in a different colour.

HINT 1: The first feeling starts with the letter 'W' and the last feeling ends in the letter 'R'.

HINT 2: The three pictures below should give you a clue to the words you are looking for!

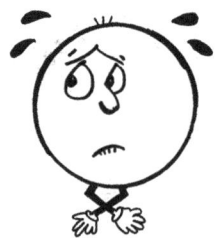 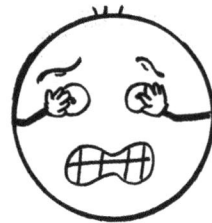 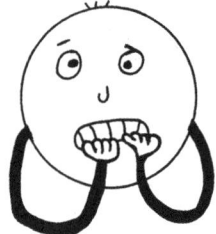

O	U	S	N
V	O	R	E
R	W	R	S
E	N	Y	S
R	A	E	F

The three feelings that you were looking for were:

Worry
For example, feeling worried if someone we care about is ill or injured.

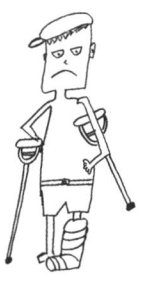

Nervousness
For example, feeling nervous when you are about to take a spelling test.

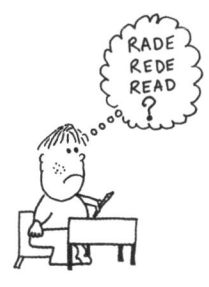

Fear
For example, feeling afraid of the dark.

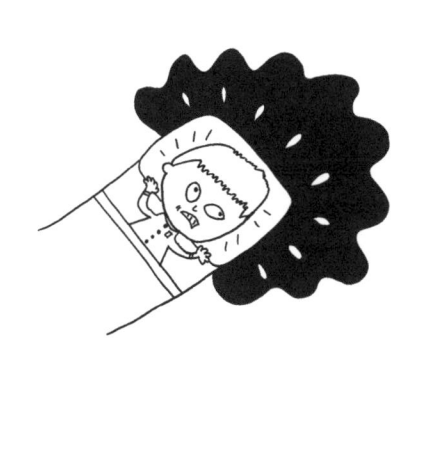

Now you know that anxiety involves the feelings of worry, nervousness and fear, let's learn more about them! In order to do that we need to:

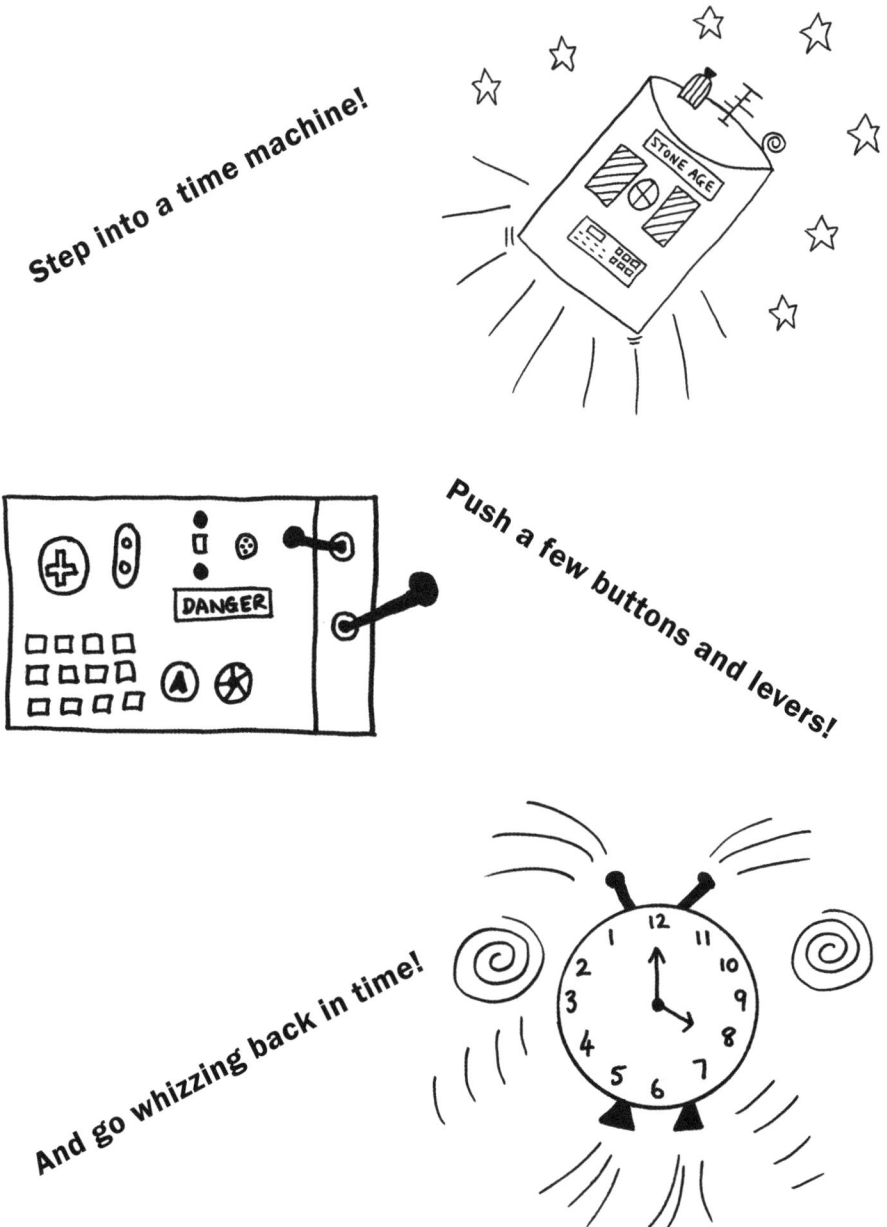

Draw your own time machine whizzing through space and time in the box below.

My time machine

Destination – The Stone Age!

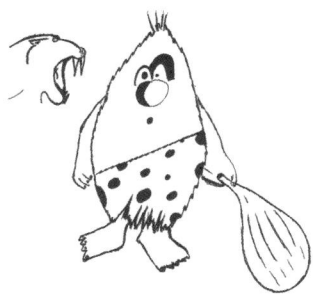

Your time machine jolts to a halt and you open the door. It is one million years ago and it's a time when cavemen and sabre-tooth tigers roam the Earth!

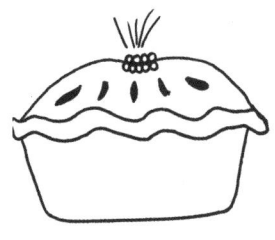

Just in front of you Caveman Colin is doing normal caveman-type things, like searching for berries to go in a caveman-sized pie for dinner!

But suddenly, you notice a scary-looking creature in the bushes behind Caveman Colin.

'It's behind you!' you shout, just like at a Christmas pantomime. At the sound of your voice, Caveman Colin turns and comes nose to nose with a sabre-tooth tiger!

Caveman Colin thinks...

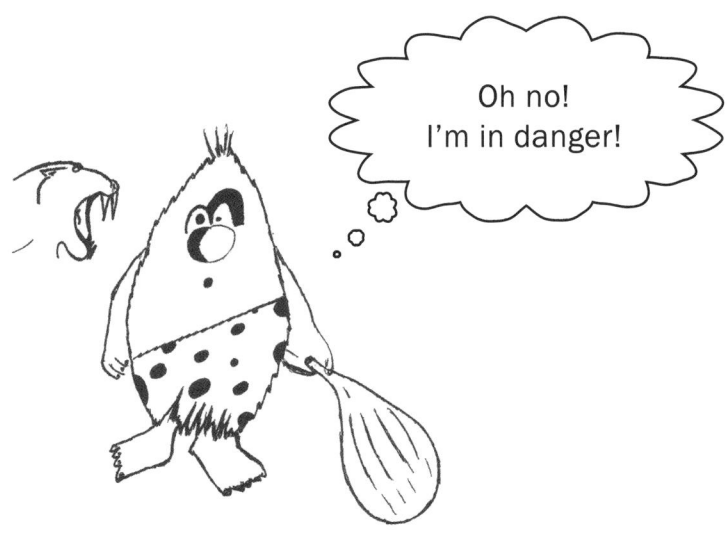

QUESTION: Which of the following do you think Caveman Colin might be feeling at this time? Colour in the face that matches your answer.

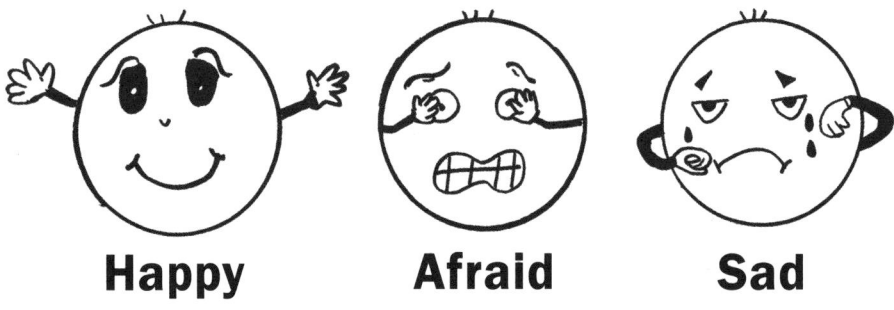

Happy **Afraid** **Sad**

Well done if you answered 'afraid'. You are correct.

And this fear sets off a warning alarm in Caveman Colin's body, just like smoke setting off a smoke alarm.

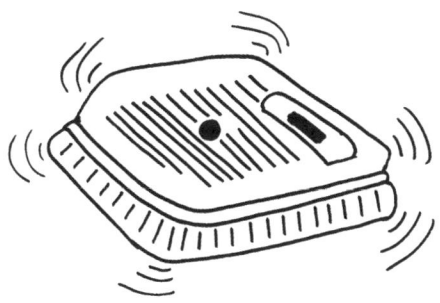

And this warning alarm causes changes in his body that will allow him to:

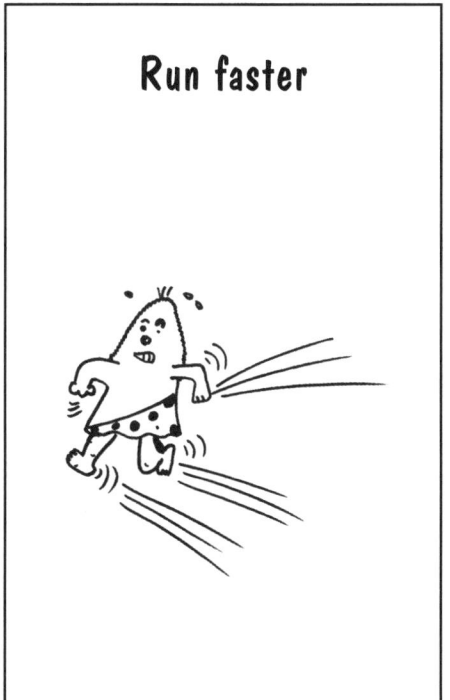

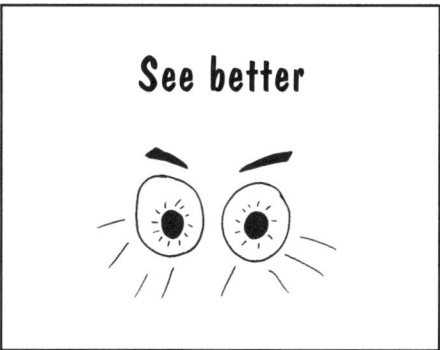

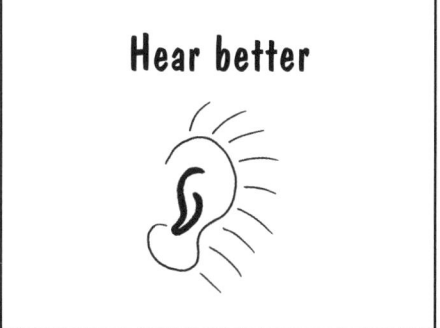

Think faster 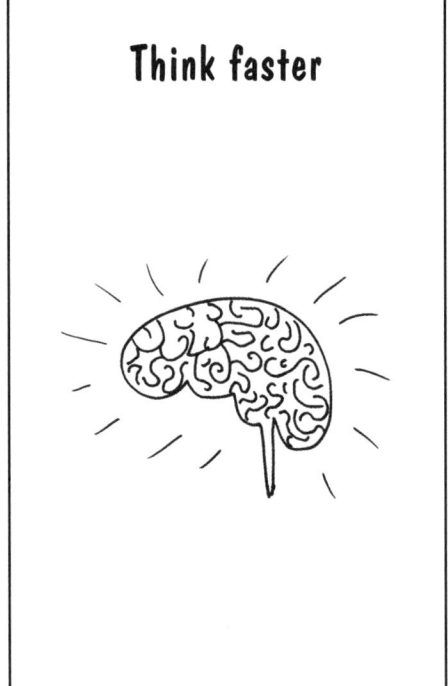	**Jump higher** 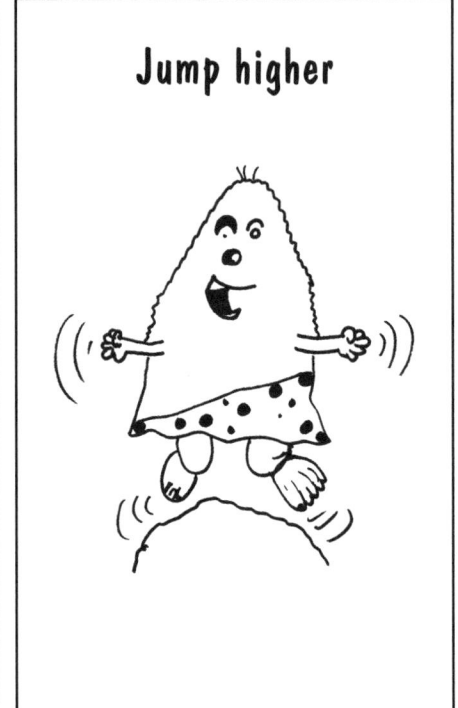
Defend self easier 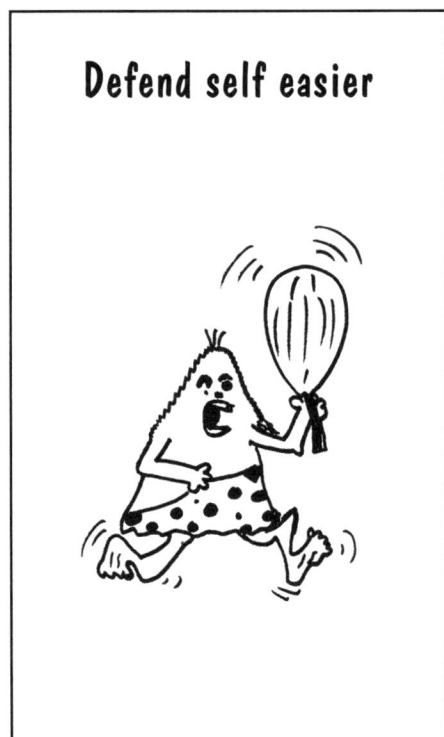	**Heal any injuries quicker** 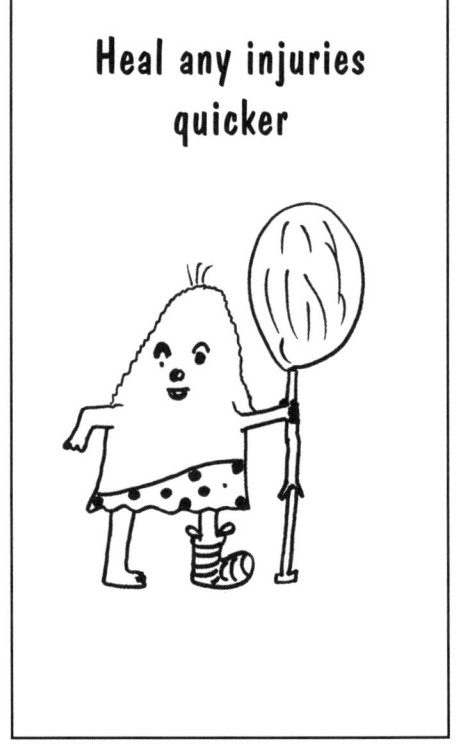

All together, these bodily changes protect Caveman Colin, just like a suit of armour. This protection will help Caveman Colin to survive the meeting with the sabre-tooth tiger by...

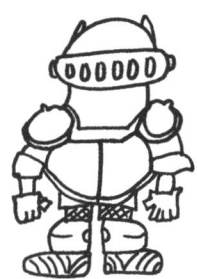

Defending himself

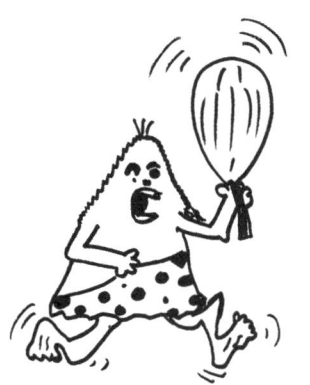
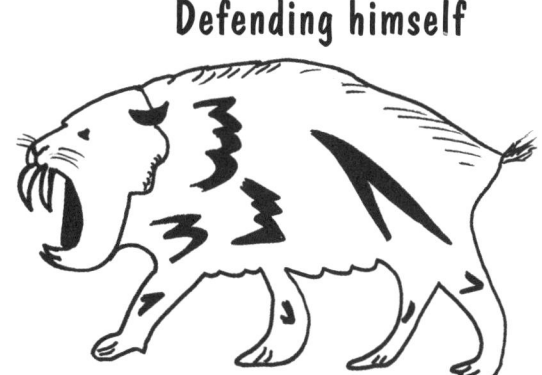

Or...

Running away to safety

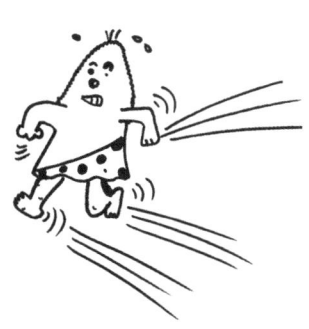
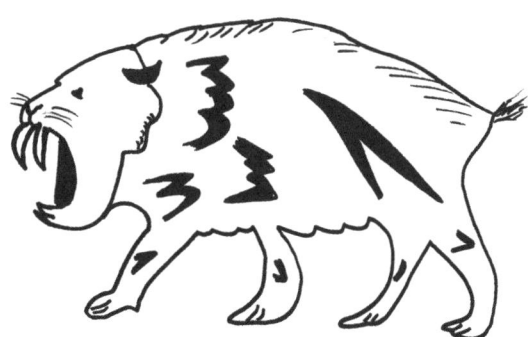

This protection is called the...

fight or flight response.

Once Caveman Colin had protected himself from the danger of the sabre-tooth tiger, he no longer needed to be afraid and his body went back to normal.

Draw your own picture of a caveman in the box below and give him a name!

My caveman's name is . . . .

Back to the Present Day

It's time to say goodbye to Caveman Colin. So jump back into your time machine! Draw the inside of your time machine in the box on the next page.

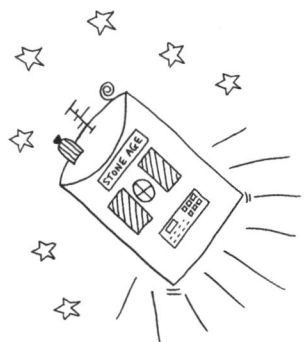

The inside of my time machine

Press some more buttons and levers in your time machine. But on this occasion, let's fly forward in time to the present day!

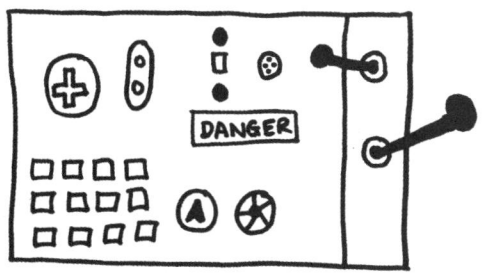

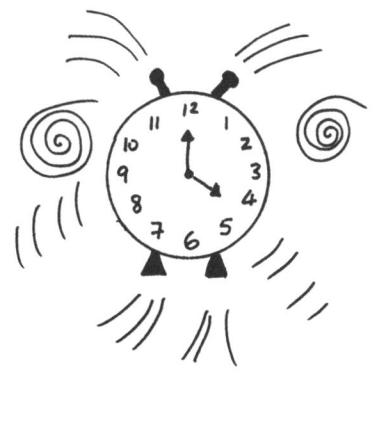

In today's world, sabre-tooth tigers are extinct. But we all still get afraid, worried or nervous sometimes in life. And when we do, a warning alarm is set off in our bodies and we have the same changes in our bodies as Caveman Colin had.

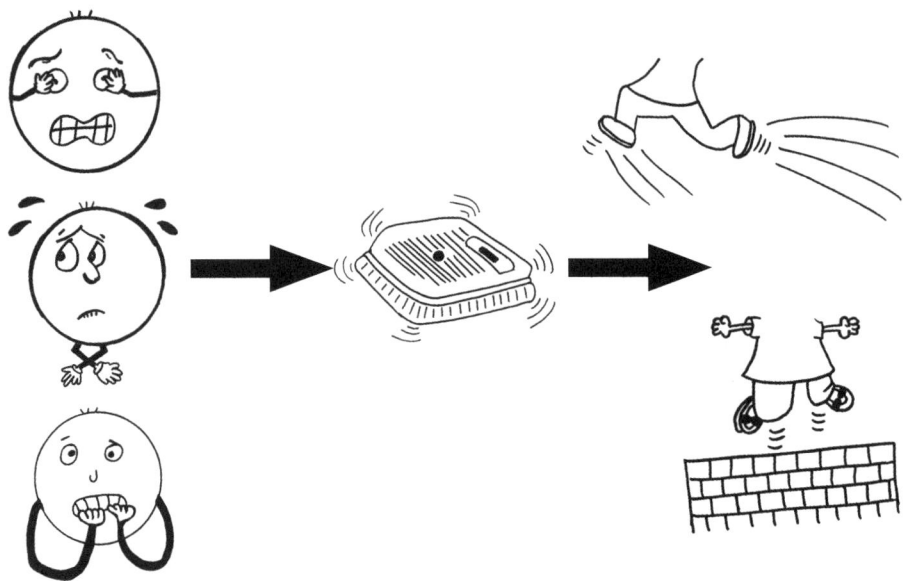

For example, Cassie, aged six, feels afraid the first time she meets a dog. But her fight or flight response stops when she realises that the dog is very friendly. Heather, aged five, feels worried the first time she goes into a swimming pool. But her fight or flight response stops when she realises that her armbands keep her afloat! Phillip, aged eight, gets nervous before his school spelling test. But his fight or flight response stops when he realises that it's quite easy.

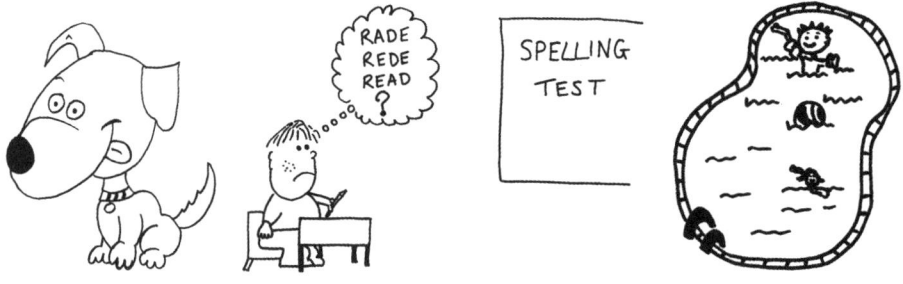

Write a story or draw a cartoon in the box on the next page called 'When Phillip was nervous before his spelling test' that shows how Phillip feels at first and then how he calms down. I've started the story off for you!

When Phillip was nervous before his spelling test

It's Friday morning and for Phillip that means school spelling test time!

As Phillip sits down in his chair, Mrs Bell, his teacher, says, 'I hope you all practised at home as your weekly spelling test is about to begin!'

Phillip feels…

But What if Your Warning Alarm Is Too Sensitive?

It is normal to feel afraid, worried or nervous and to go through the fight or flight response sometimes. But some people get worried, nervous or afraid a lot and their bodies go through the fight or flight response too often. When this happens we call it...

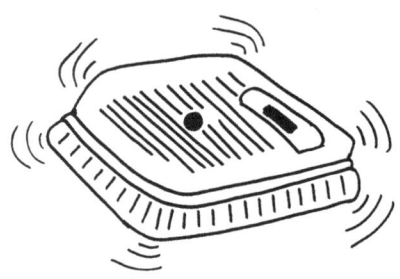

anxiety!

And when you experience anxiety you can...

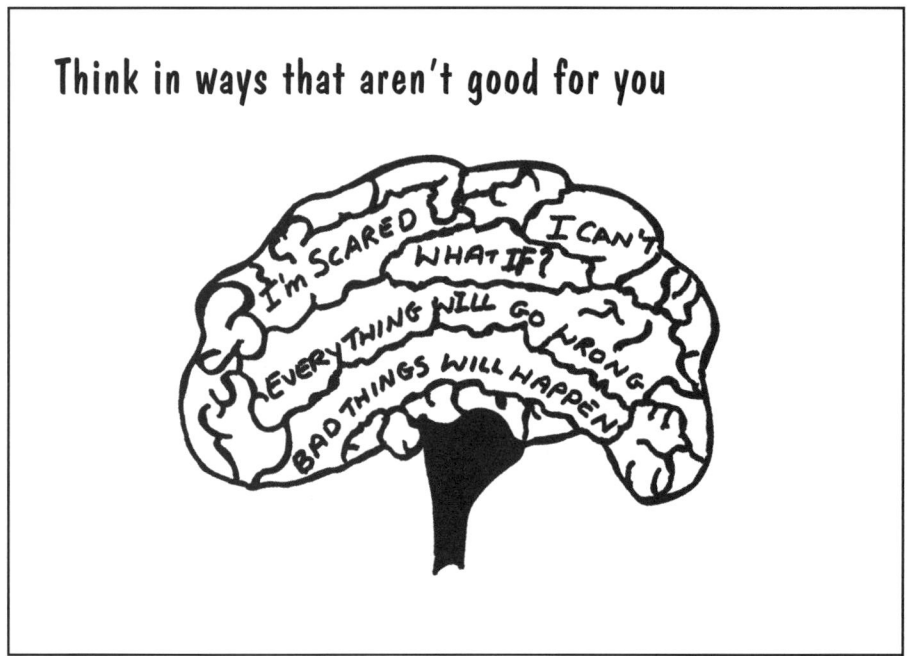

Have physical feelings in your body that aren't good for you

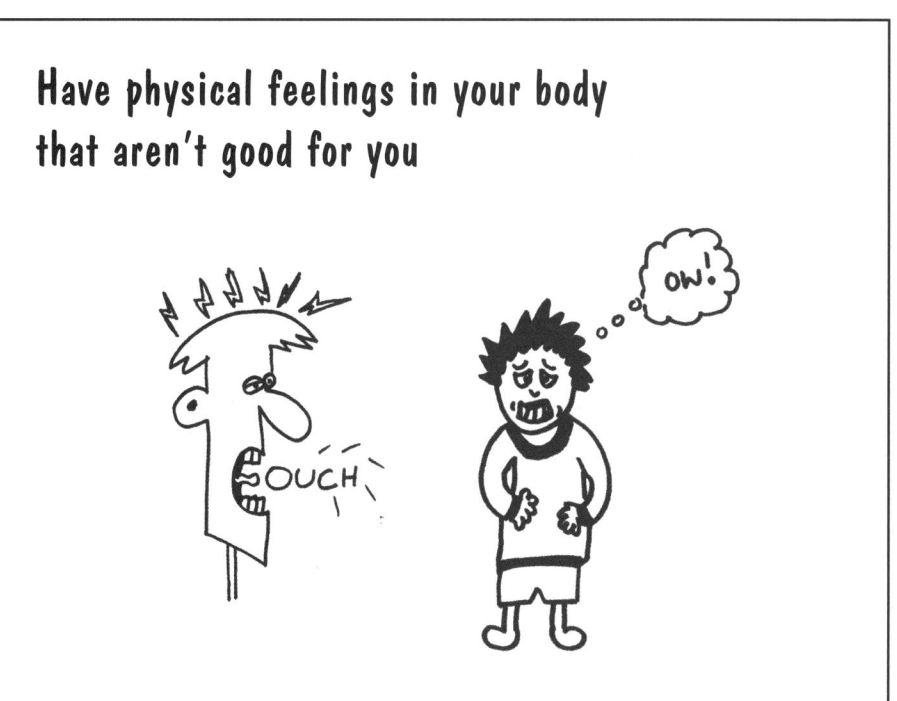

Act in ways that aren't good for you

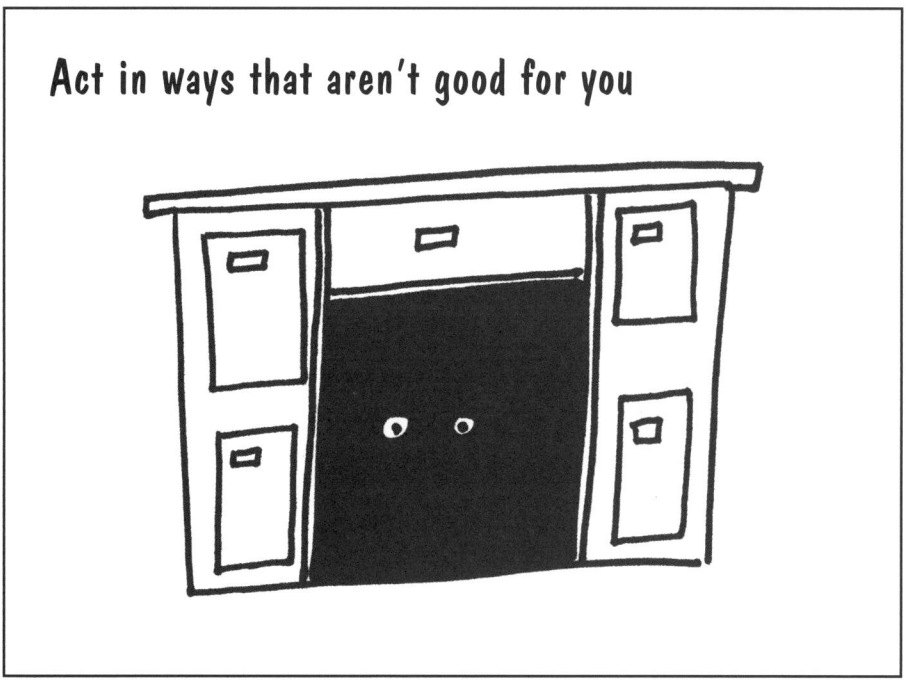

You will learn about all of these aspects of anxiety and why some people get anxious and others don't as you work through this book. But before you do, give yourself a big clap for completing Step 3 in starving your Anxiety Gremlin and colour in your third **Starving the Anxiety Gremlin Star**! Well done! You are doing brilliantly!

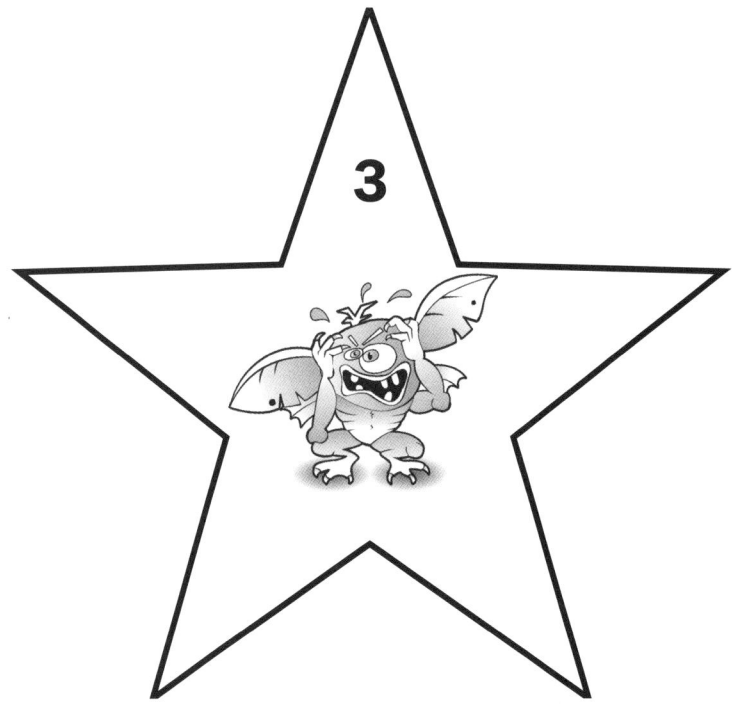

Now complete one or both of the following **Just for Fun Puzzles** as a reward for all you've learnt! Enjoy!

Go Dotty!

Join up the dots on the following page to reveal a picture. Start with dot number 1 and finish with dot number 90. Then why not colour in the picture when you have finished?

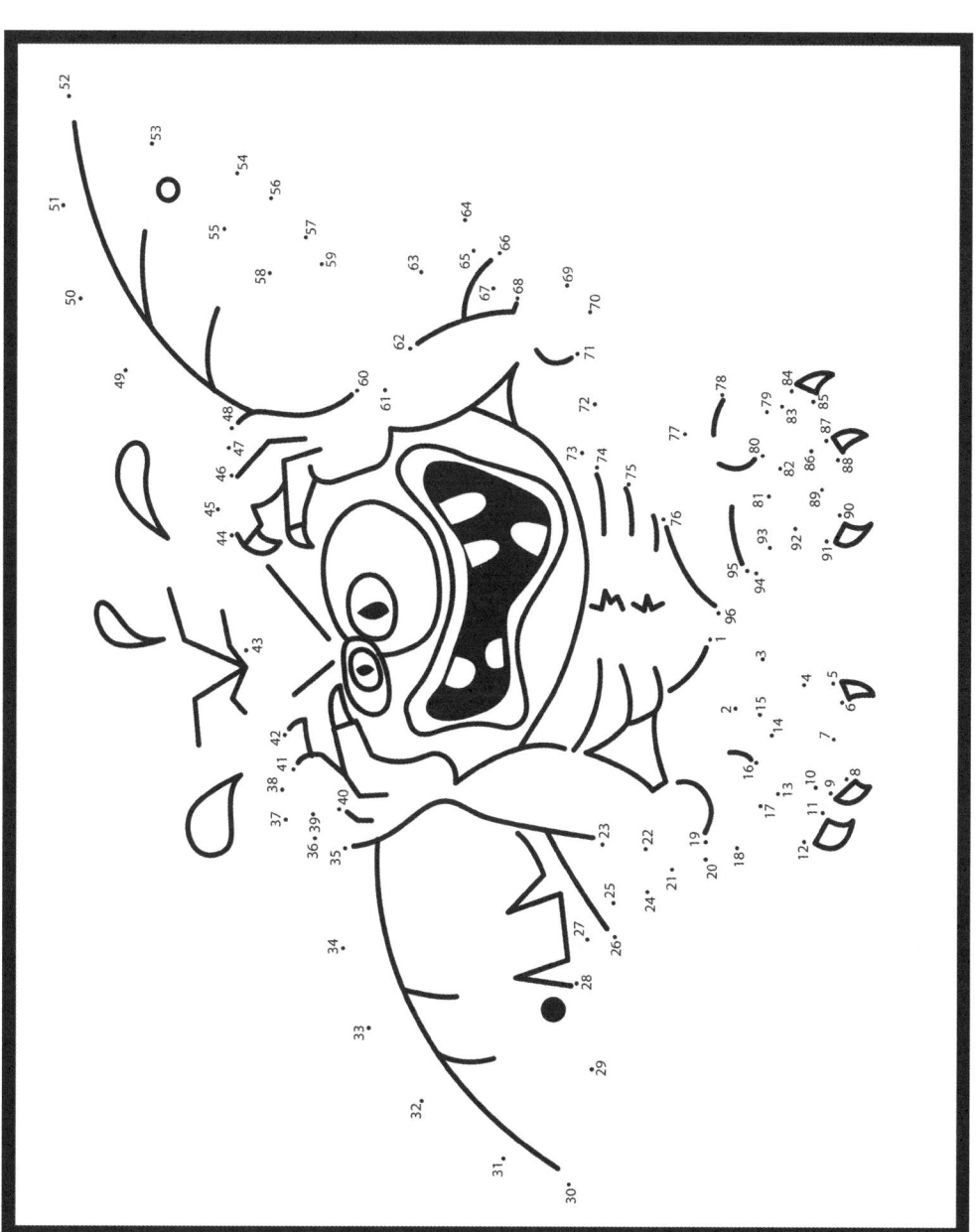

Word Hunt

How many times can you find the word 'anxiety' in the face below?

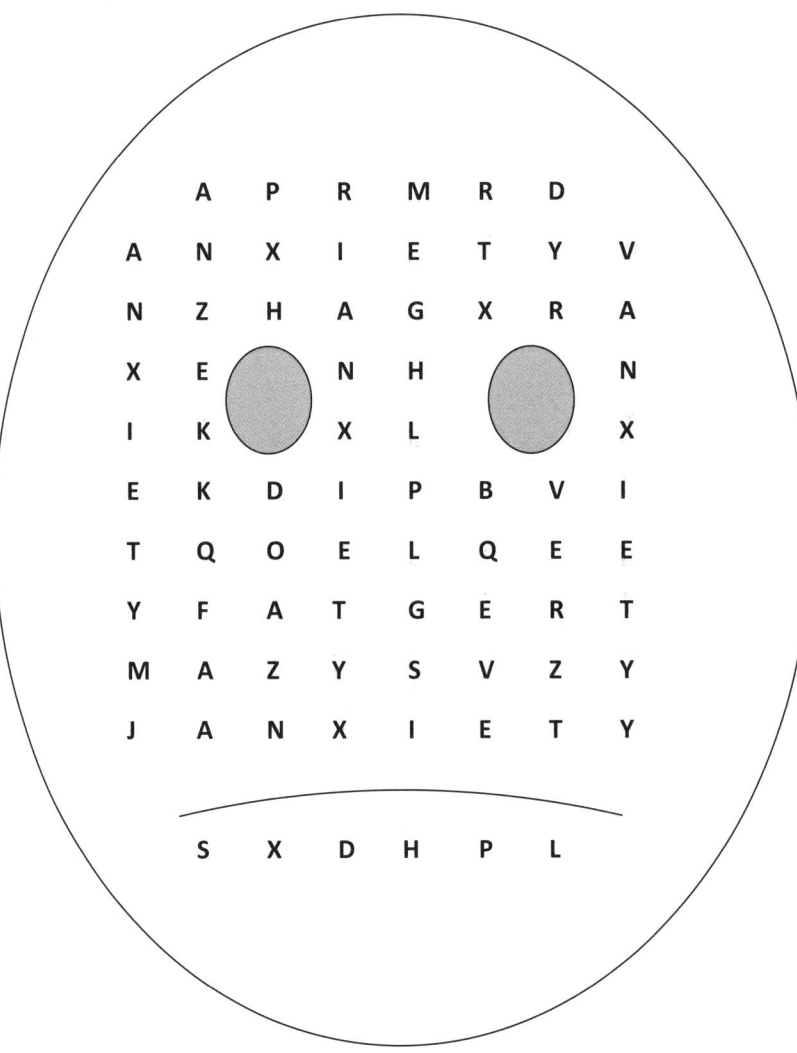

I can find the word 'anxiety' _____ times.

5
Things We Get Anxious About

Step 4 in your mission to starve your Anxiety Gremlin is to learn about anxiety triggers.

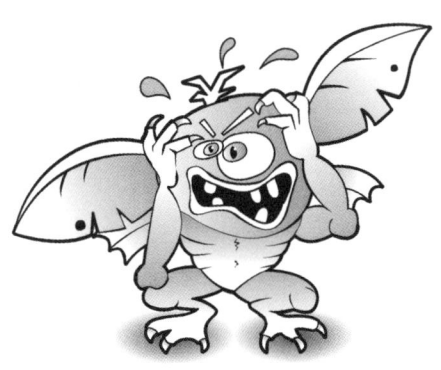

Anxiety Triggers

When we feel anxious it is often in response to something that we call a...

trigger.

Anxiety triggers can be:

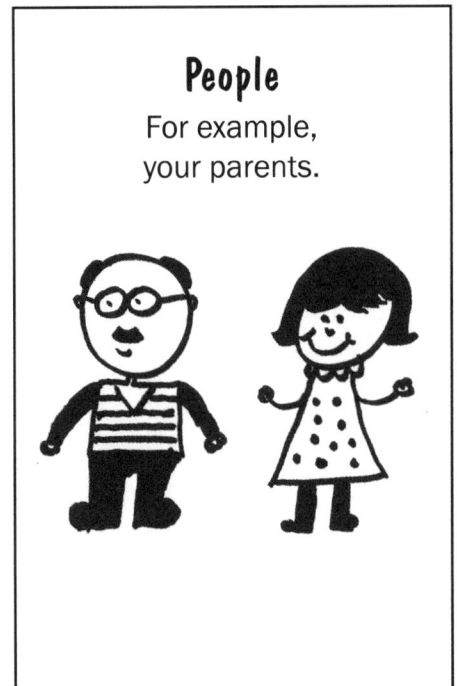

People
For example, your parents.

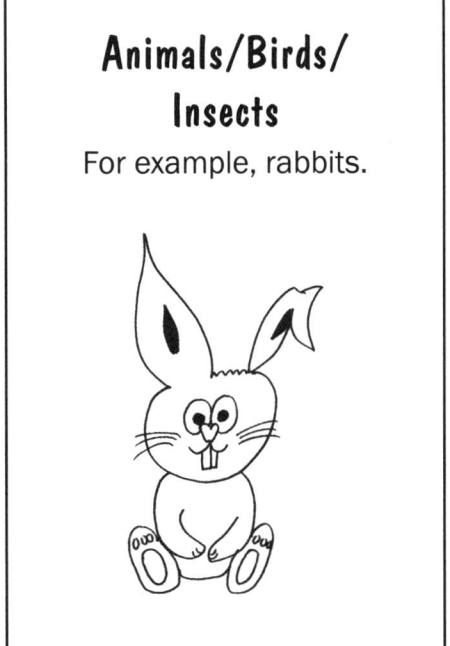

Animals/Birds/Insects
For example, rabbits.

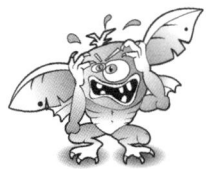 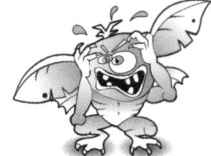 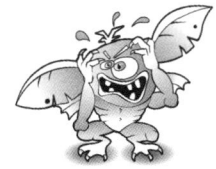

Someone's actions
For example, bullying.

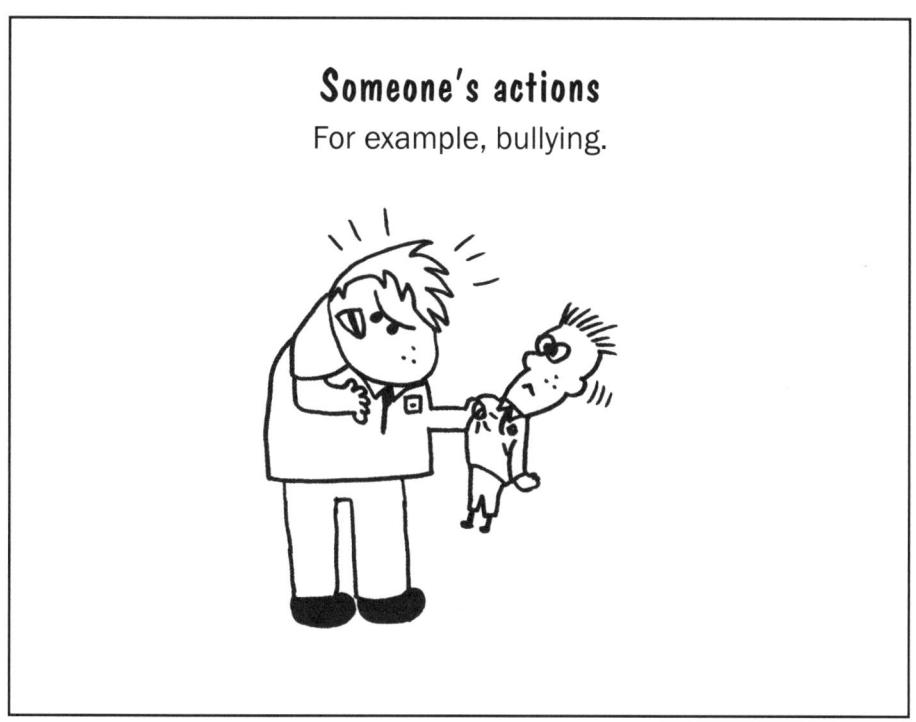

Places
For example, school.

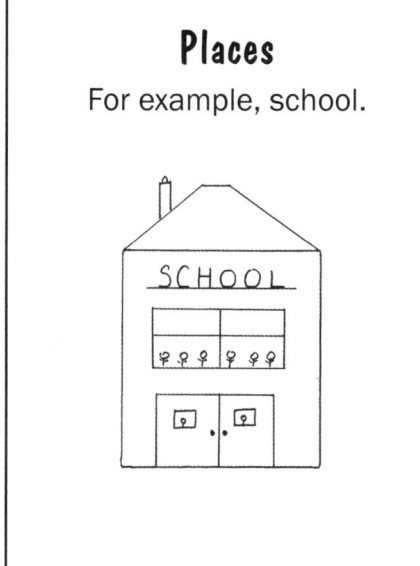

Situations
For example, reading aloud in class.

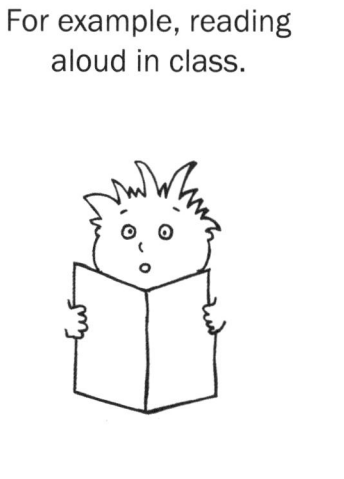

Your Anxiety Triggers

Write down or draw the types of people, animals, birds, insects, places, situations or people's actions that you often get anxious about in the box below. If it is easier for you, why not talk to an adult about this or cut pictures out of magazines and comics and make a poster of the things that you get anxious about?

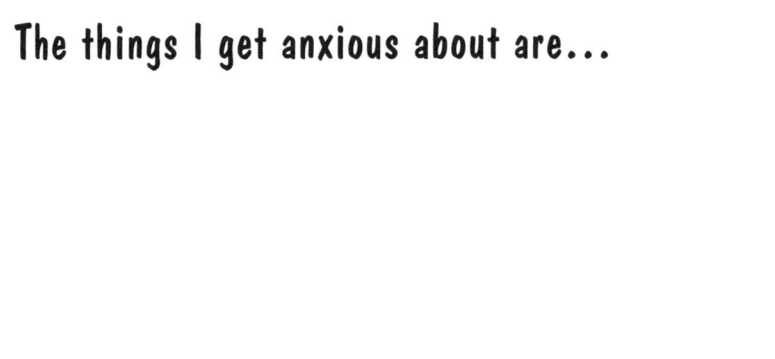

The things I get anxious about are...

Everyone's Anxiety Is Different

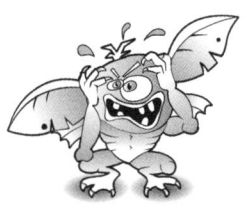

Some people get anxious about one particular thing, other people get anxious about a few things and some people get anxious about lots of different things.

Here are some stories about other children and what they get anxious about to show you how we are all different.

Things We Get Anxious About

Max is seven years old and he worries all the time about something bad happening to his parents when he is not with them.

Fiona is seven years old. She once vomited during a school assembly because she had a tummy bug. She now worries every week about whether she will vomit again during assembly.

Sally is six years old and she is afraid of spiders. She worries everywhere she goes in case she sees a spider.

Abdul is eight years old. He is afraid of going to the doctor.

Ben is nine years old and he is afraid of certain foods.

Melissa is five years old and she is afraid of thunderstorms. She worries about going to school every day in case there is a thunderstorm when she is there.

Greg is eight years old. He watched a cartoon about ghosts and now he worries all the time about whether there is one in his house.

Tim is eight years old and he is afraid of the dark.

Helen is nine years old and she worries all the time about catching germs and getting poorly.

Grace is six years old and she is afraid of leaving the house.

Wesley is seven years old and is afraid of heights.

Carla is nine years old and she worries all the time about going to the toilet in other people's houses.

Mandy is eight years old and she worries all the time about making mistakes in school.

Neela is eight years old and she is afraid of dogs.

Nicholas is six years old and he worries every day that his mum will forget to pick him up from school.

David is seven years old and he worries that the other children at school don't like him and will laugh at him.

Freddie is eight years old and he worries that bad things will happen if he doesn't put his pencils back in a certain order in his pencil case and if his teddies aren't in a certain order in his room.

Lucy is nine years old. She worries every time she sees or hears the number ten in case it means something bad will happen.

Find the Pairs!

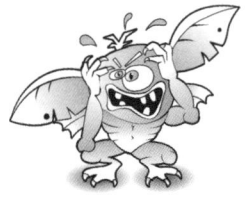

Now you have read all the children's stories, I have a puzzle for you to complete. Below are lots of pictures that represent all the things that the children were anxious about in the stories that you have just read. See if you can match up the right child with the right picture! Write the child's name under the picture. I've started one for you!

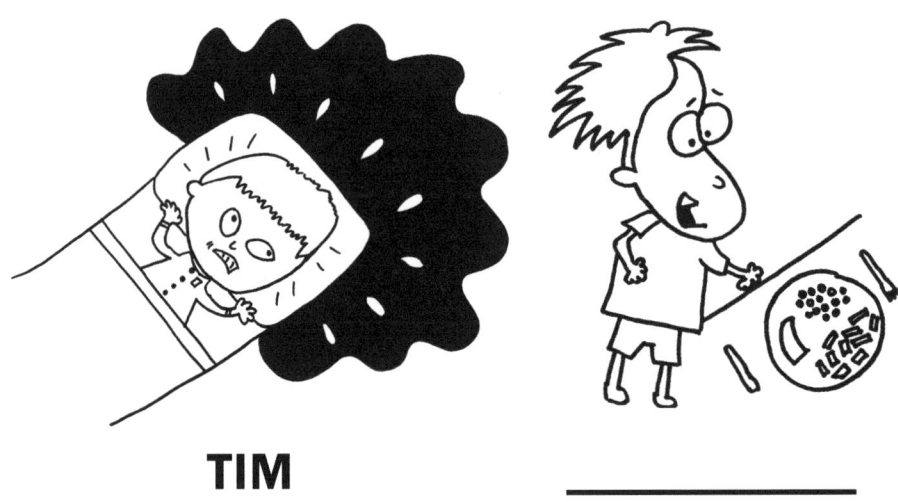

TIM

_____

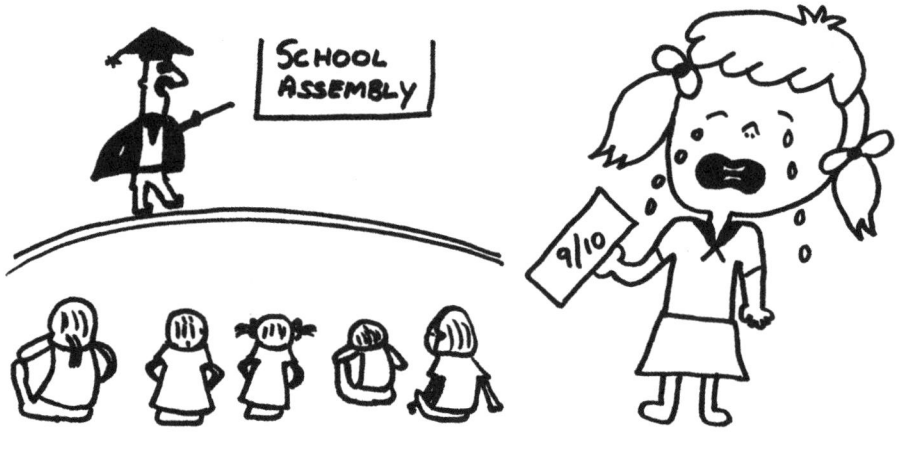

_____   _____

Things We Get Anxious About 65

SCHOOL

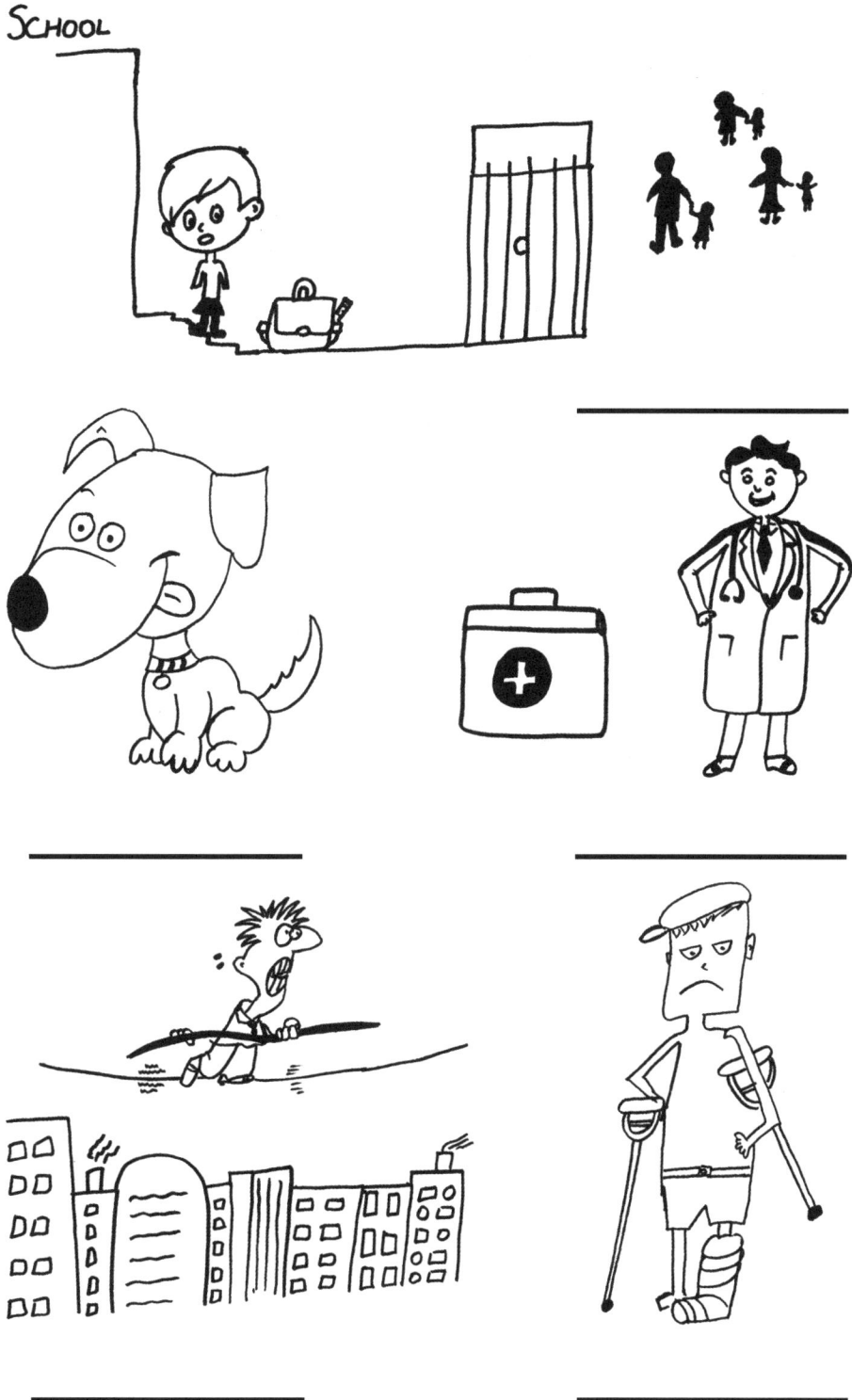

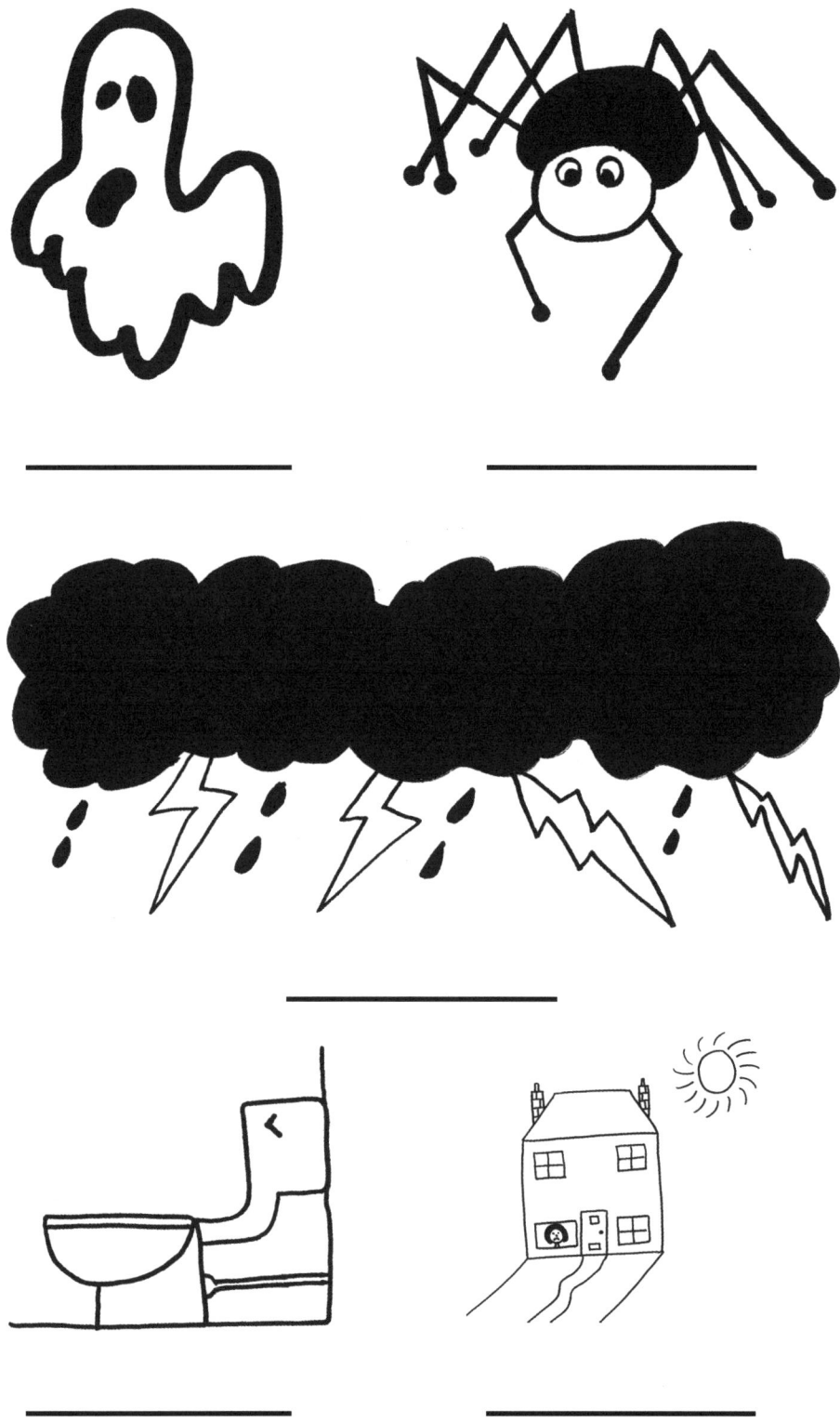

Things We Get Anxious About   67

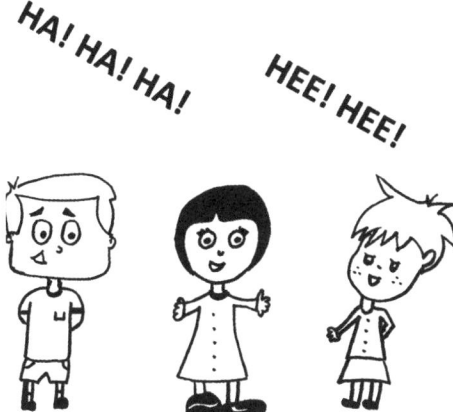 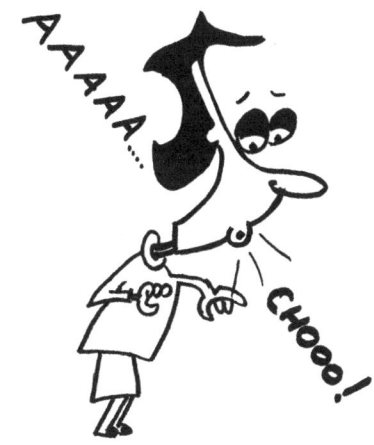

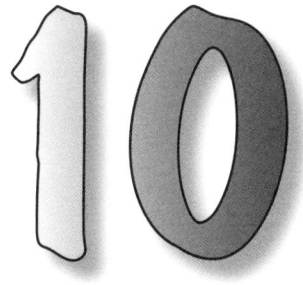 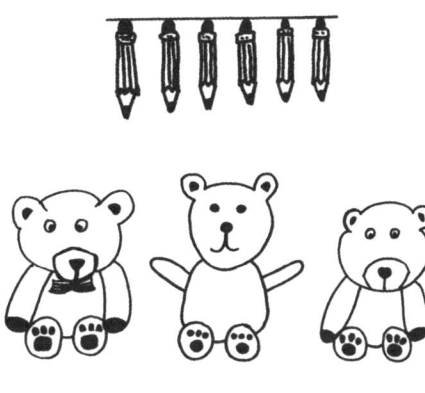

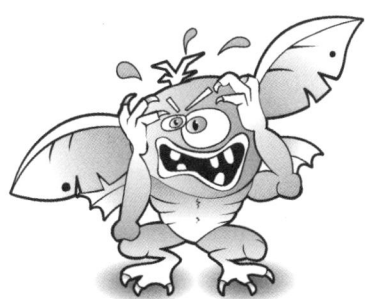 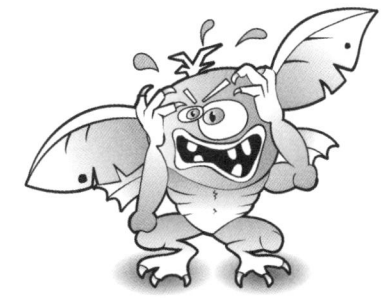

Congratulations! You've completed Step 4 in starving your Anxiety Gremlin. You've learnt lots about anxiety and you're doing really well! Be proud and colour in your fourth **Starving the Anxiety Gremlin Star**!

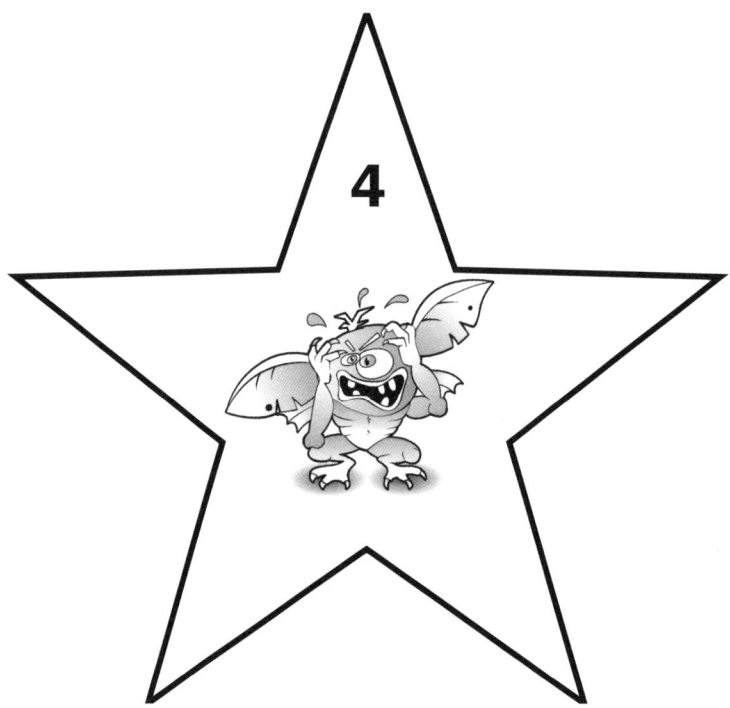

Now complete one or both of the following **Just for Fun Puzzles** as a reward for all your hard work! Enjoy!

How Many Gremlins?

There are lots of Anxiety Gremlin pictures in this chapter. See how many you can find and write your answer below.

There are _____ Anxiety Gremlins in this chapter.

Odd Gremlin Out

Look at the pictures below and see if you can work out which Anxiety Gremlin is the odd gremlin out.

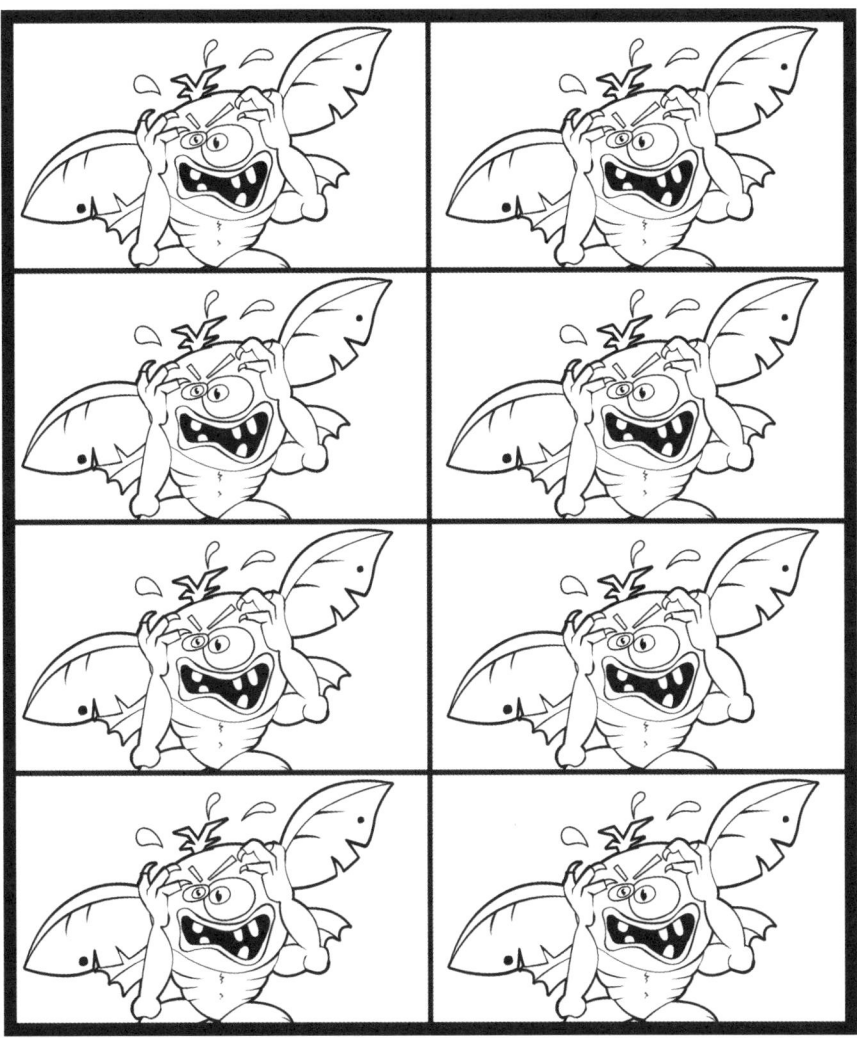

6

Why We Get Anxious

Step 5 in your mission to starve your Anxiety Gremlin is to learn why we get anxious.

Who or What Makes Us Anxious?

In the last chapter you learnt that we all get anxious about different things. What one child gets anxious about, another child may feel completely different about. Let's look at why this is by learning about two seven-year-old girls called Debbie and Joanne.

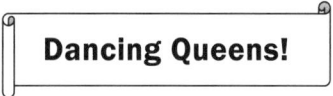
Dancing Queens!

Debbie and Joanne are best friends and they both love to dance! Their mums are professional dancers. Debbie and Joanne dream of having jobs as dancers one day so they can be just like their mums.

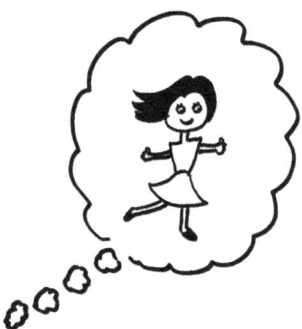

Debbie and Joanne beg their mums to sign them up for dance classes. So their mums take them along to a class to see what it is like. Debbie and Joanne watch the other children dancing together and having lots of fun.

On the way home, Joanne says, 'I can't wait to go to class next week! It's going to be so much fun!' But Debbie says nothing.

All week Joanne is excited and talks about nothing but the dance class. 'I'm looking forward to meeting all the other children,'

Joanne thinks to herself. 'They were really great dancers. I can't wait to learn how to be as good as them!'

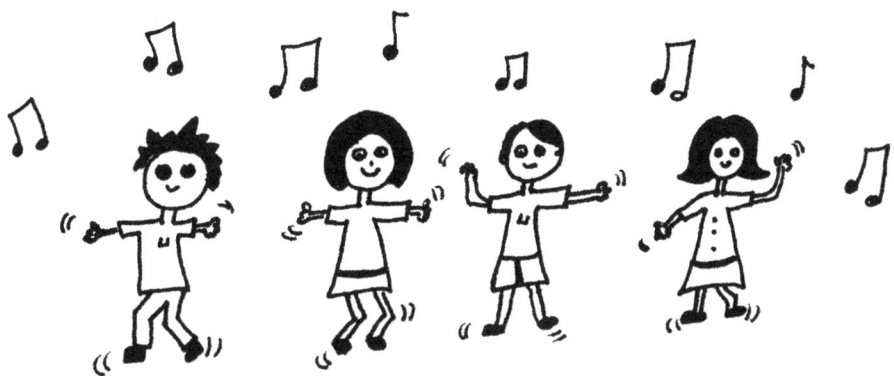

But seeing all the other children dancing so well has had a different effect on Debbie. 'I'm never going to be as good as those other children,' Debbie thinks to herself all week. 'I'm going to make a fool of myself when I dance in front of the other children and they will all laugh at me. Then I'll never be able to go back to the class and I'll never become a professional dancer when I'm older.'

Debbie struggles to get to sleep every night as all the thoughts about the dance class whizz round and round in her head and the night before the class she has a really bad nightmare. But Debbie doesn't tell her mum how she is feeling.

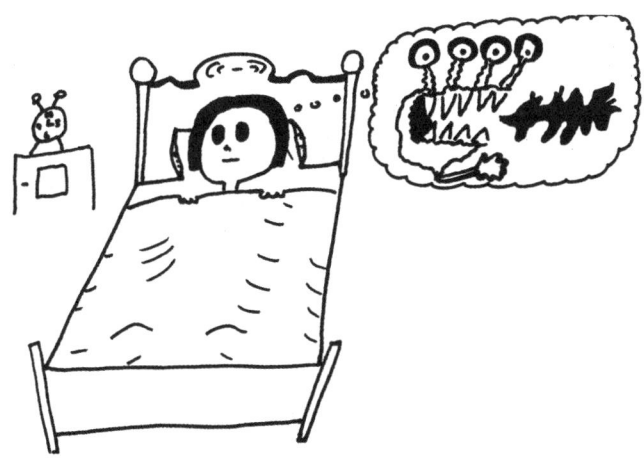

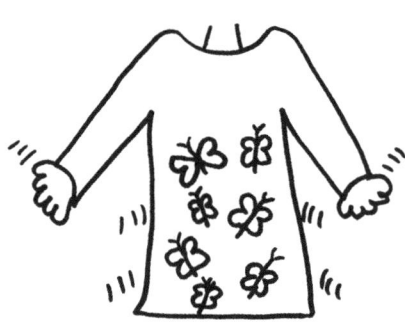

The day of the class arrives and Debbie feels sick and has butterflies in her tummy, but once again she keeps her worries to herself. 'My mum will be disappointed in me and won't love me as much if I tell her I can't go to dance class,' thinks Debbie. So she gets into the car with her mum and they go to pick up Joanne and her mum.

'I can't wait to get there,' says Joanne as she climbs into the car.

They arrive at the dance class and make their way to the dance hall. Joanne dances her way through the door with a big grin on her face.

'Hello everyone!' she shouts to the other children.

But Debbie stops at the door and bursts into tears. 'I can't go in, Mum. I'm sorry, but I can't. I'm too scared. I'm scared I'll be useless and all the other children with laugh at me.'

Debbie's mum bends down and gives her daughter a big hug.

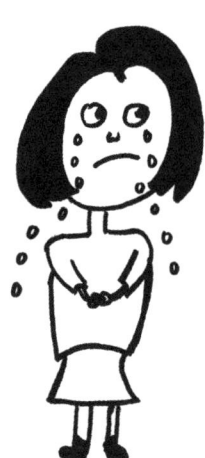

The End!

QUESTION: Who made Debbie anxious? Circle your answer.

The children in the dance class   Debbie   Debbie's mum

When answering this question, a lot of people (including many adults) would say the children in the dance class. But the answer is Debbie! Let's look at why.

Do you remember the anxiety **triggers** that we looked at in the last chapter? Here's a reminder!

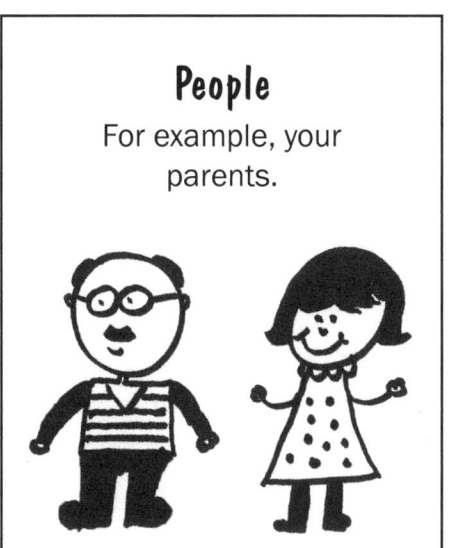

People
For example, your parents.

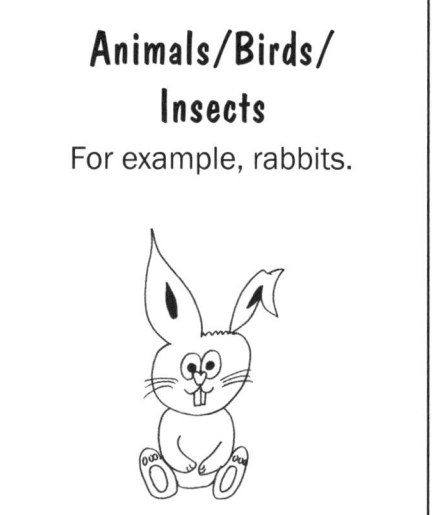

Animals/Birds/Insects
For example, rabbits.

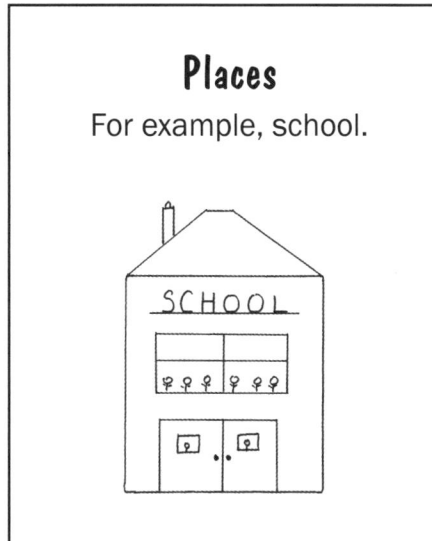

Places
For example, school.

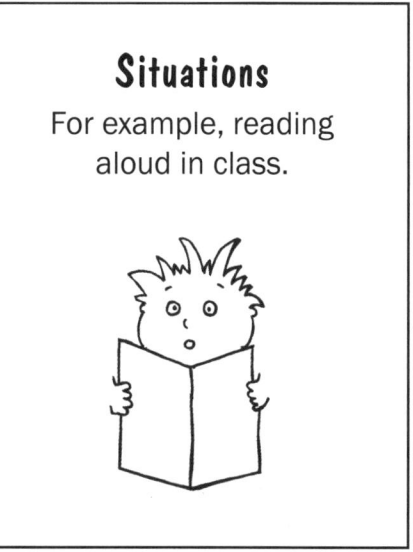

Situations
For example, reading aloud in class.

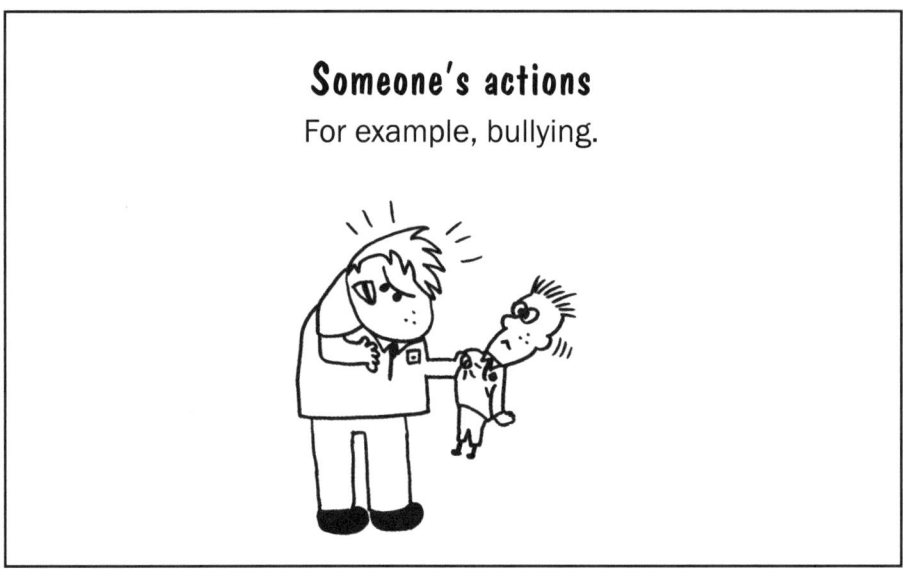

Someone's actions
For example, bullying.

People often think that these things **make** us anxious.

But they don't.

You see it's not the person, the animal, the bird, the insect, the place, the situation or someone's actions that makes you anxious. If it was, we would all feel and act in the same way in the same situations.

But we don't.

Think about Debbie and Joanne for a moment.

- Both girls had mums who used to be dancers.
- Both girls dreamed of getting a job as a dancer when they were older.
- Both girls joined the same dance class.
- Both girls watched the same children dancing at the dance class.
- Debbie got anxious but Joanne didn't.

QUESTION: Why do you think Debbie got anxious but Joanne didn't?

To help you answer that question, write how Debbie and Joanne were thinking about the dance class in the thought bubbles on the next page.

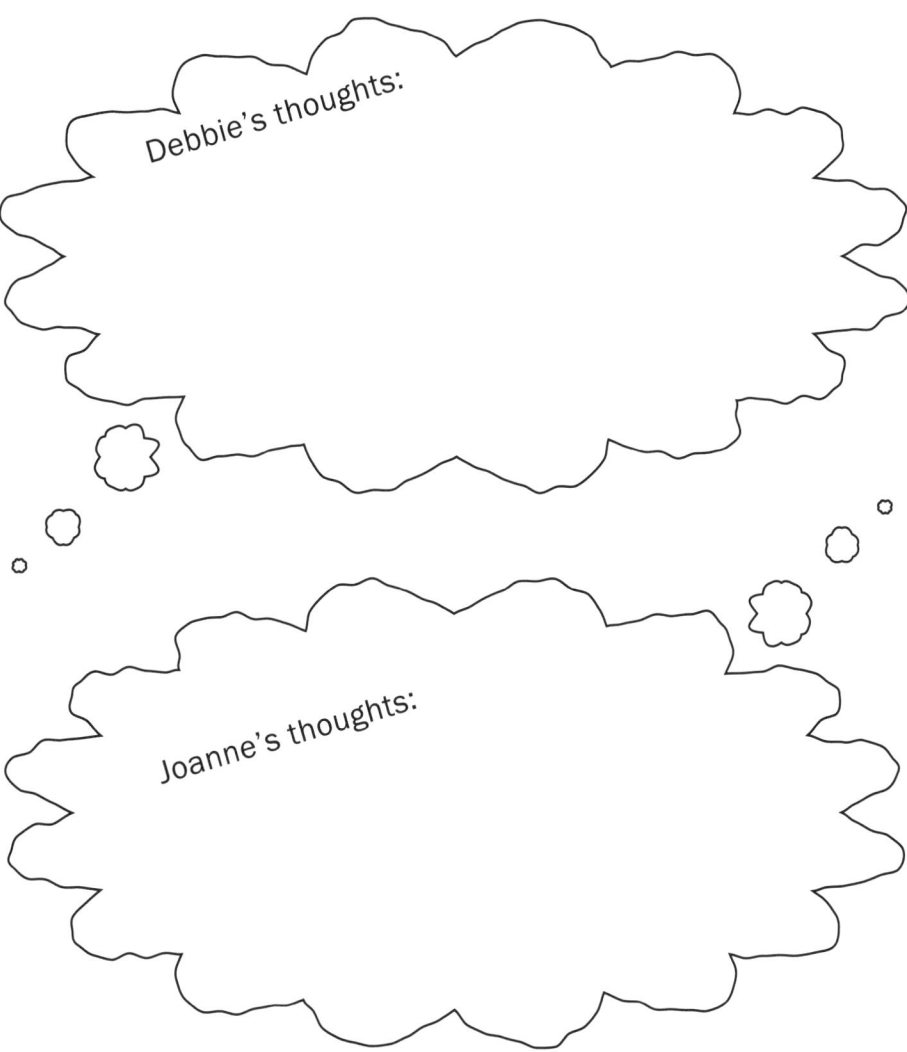

Debbie and Joanne were thinking differently from each other. This is why Debbie got anxious but Joanne didn't. So what does this show us about why we get anxious?

Why Do We Get Anxious?

We get anxious because of...

how we think!

Let's look at another example that shows this...

Imagine that you've just moved to a new school and at the end of the first week one of the children in your class invites you to their birthday party.

THOUGHTS A

You might think...

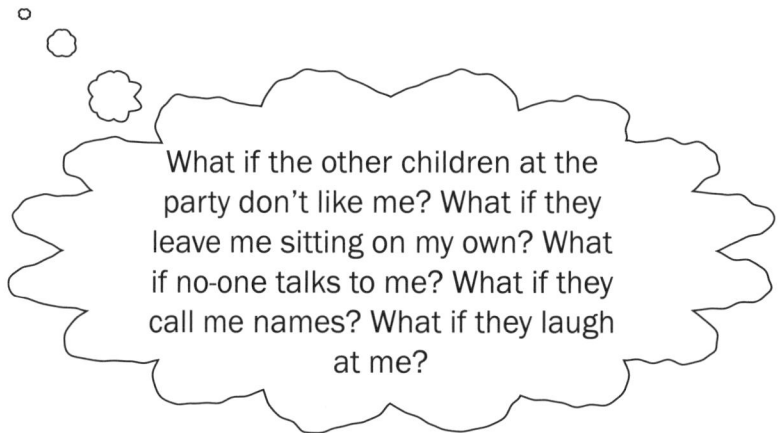

What if the other children at the party don't like me? What if they leave me sitting on my own? What if no-one talks to me? What if they call me names? What if they laugh at me?

QUESTION: If you were thinking those thoughts, how anxious would you be? Circle your answer.

Very anxious   Anxious   Not very anxious

THOUGHTS B

But what if you had the following thoughts instead?

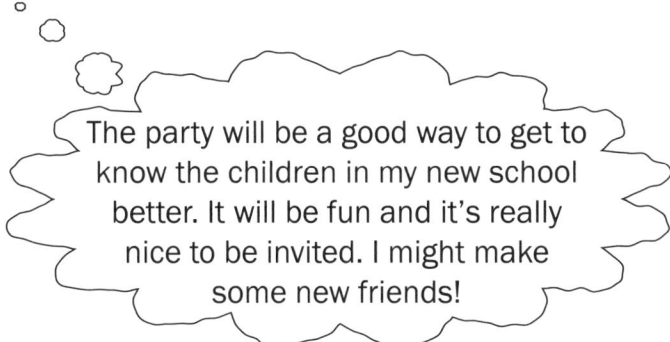

The party will be a good way to get to know the children in my new school better. It will be fun and it's really nice to be invited. I might make some new friends!

QUESTION: Now how anxious do you think you would be? Circle your answer.

Very anxious   Anxious   Not very anxious

I bet you would be more anxious as a result of Thoughts A than Thoughts B! This is because Thoughts A were coming through your...

Anxiety Thinking Glasses!

What Are Anxiety Thinking Glasses?

There are nine types of Anxiety Thinking Glasses. You will find them all on the next few pages.

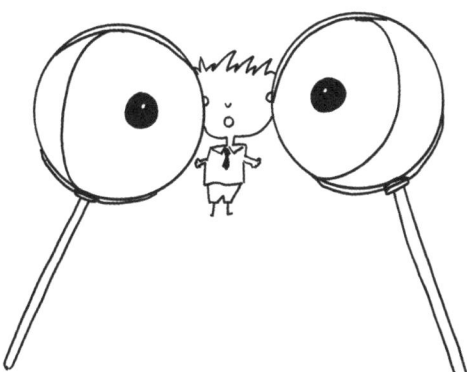

Magnifying Glasses

When you think through these glasses everything seems bigger, worse, more important or more dangerous than it actually is!

Make-Believe Glasses

When you think through these glasses you imagine things to be true even though you don't know whether they are true or not!

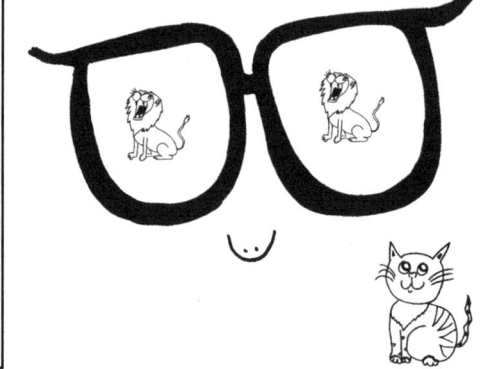

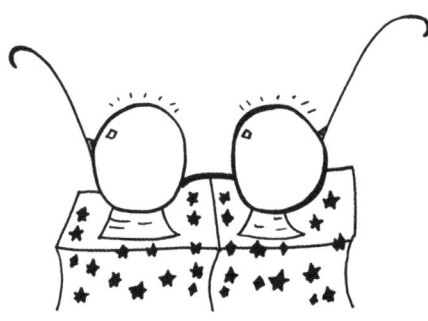

Fortune-Telling Glasses

When you think through these glasses you predict that bad things will happen in the future!

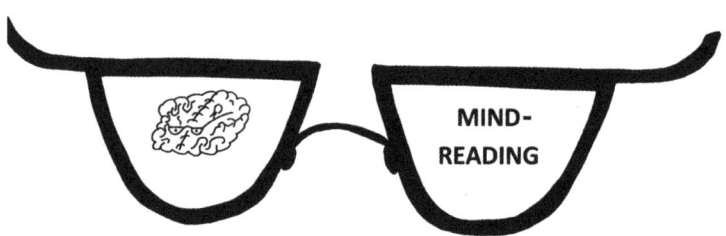

Mind-Reading Glasses

When you think through these glasses you imagine what other people are thinking even though you don't know if it's true or not!

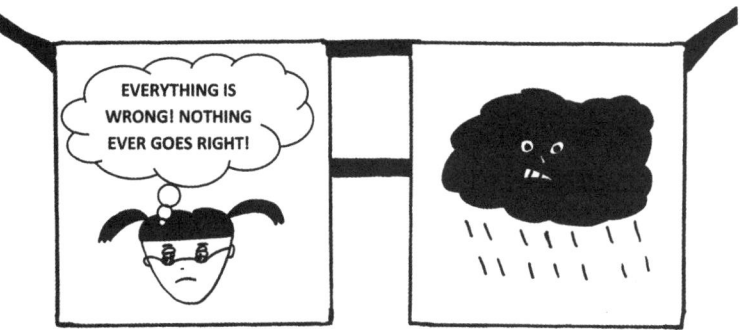

Doom and Gloom Glasses

When you think through these glasses you see the worst in everything around you and think that everything is wrong or will go wrong!

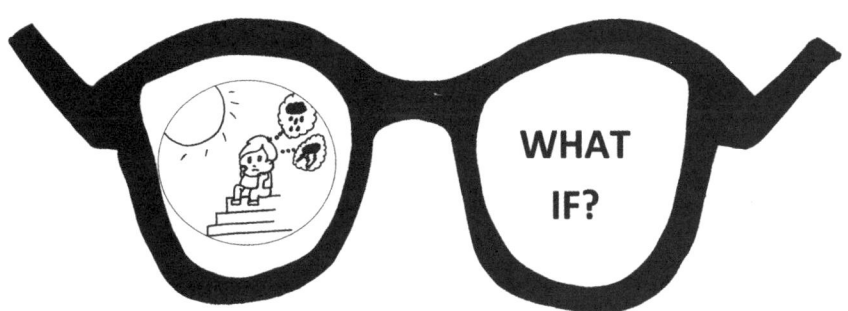

What If? Glasses

When you think through these glasses you ask yourself, 'What if this bad thing happens?' or 'What if that bad thing happens?' even though they are unlikely to happen!

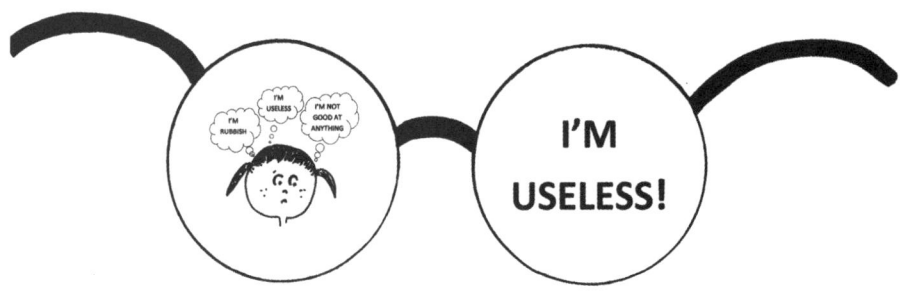

I'm Useless! Glasses
When you think through these glasses you put yourself down!

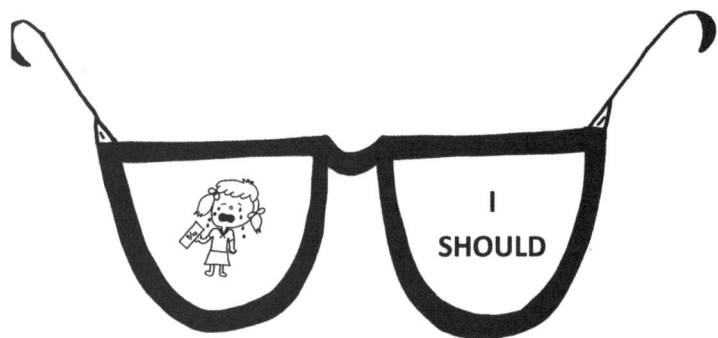

I Should Glasses
When you think through these glasses you think you should be perfect at things and not make mistakes. You also think that if you're not perfect, bad things will happen, that you're not good enough and that people won't like or love you!

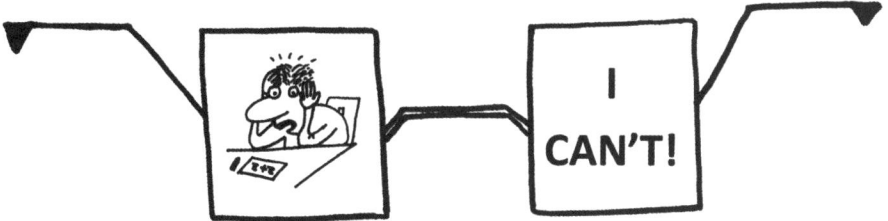

I Can't! Glasses
When you think through these glasses you think you can't do things even though you can!

Which Anxiety Thinking Glasses do you often wear? Draw a picture of yourself wearing those glasses in the box below.

Me wearing Anxiety Thinking Glasses

When we get anxious, we often think through our Anxiety Thinking Glasses. And your Anxiety Gremlin wants you to wear these all the time! Let's see why.

How Do Our Thoughts Feed the Anxiety Gremlin?

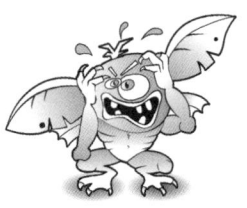

You already know that the Anxiety Gremlin is a troublesome pest whose favourite food is your anxiety, and the more anxiety you feed him, the bigger and bigger he gets! Well, one of the ways you feed him is by thinking thoughts through your Anxiety Thinking Glasses! The more you think through your Anxiety Thinking Glasses, the more you feed your Anxiety Gremlin and the bigger and bigger he gets!

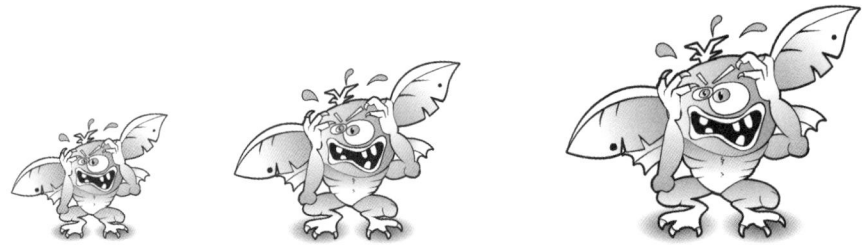

And the bigger the Anxiety Gremlin gets, the more anxious you will get.

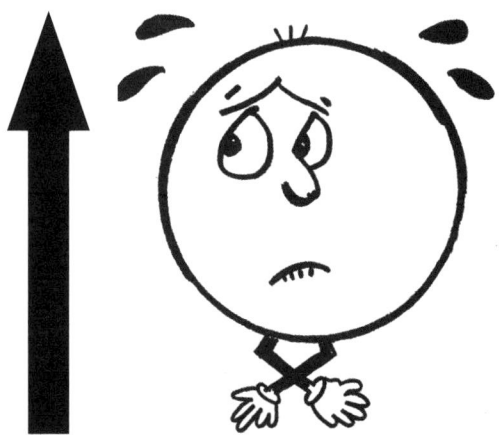

And the more anxious you get, the harder and harder it is to take your Anxiety Thinking Glasses off and anxious thoughts get stuck in your head.

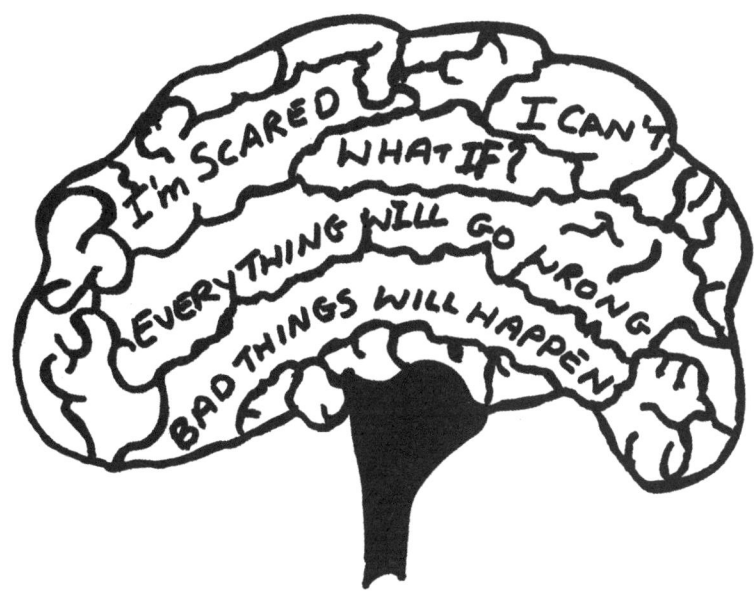

They play over and over again in your mind just like an iPod playing a song on repeat!

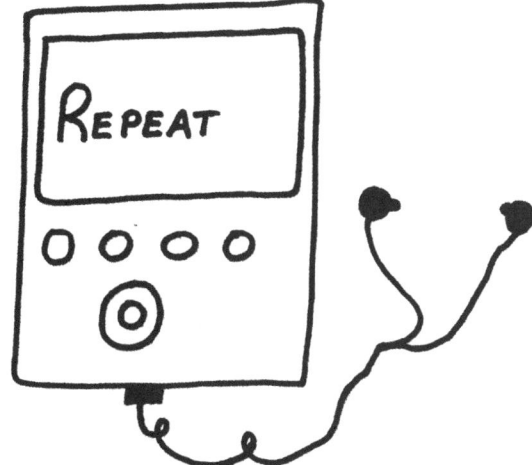

Congratulations on completing Step 5 in starving your Anxiety Gremlin. You have done so well so far! Praise yourself and colour in your fifth **Starving the Anxiety Gremlin Star**!

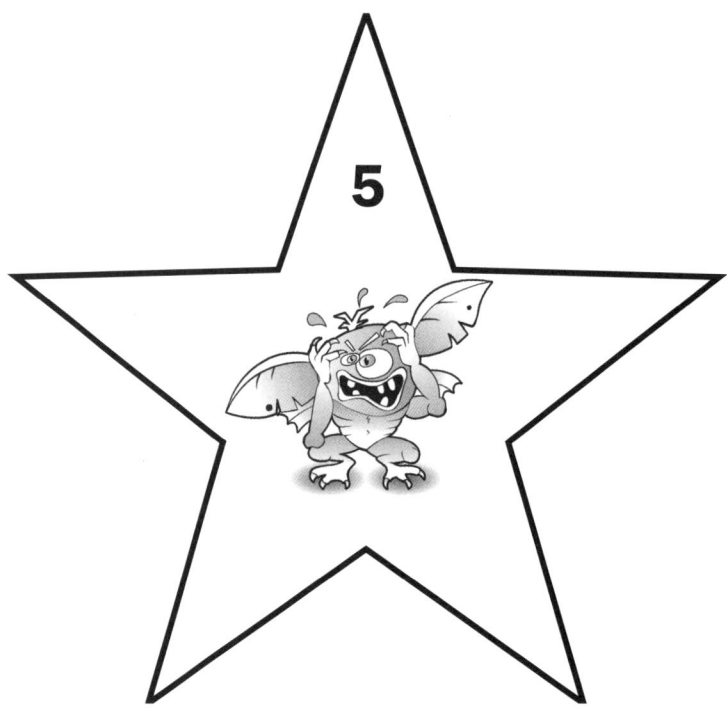

Now complete one or both of the following **Just for Fun Puzzles** as a reward for all your hard work! Have fun!

Match Four!

There are lots of pictures of Gremlins on the following page. Your task is to find four identical Anxiety Gremlins amongst them all. Good luck!

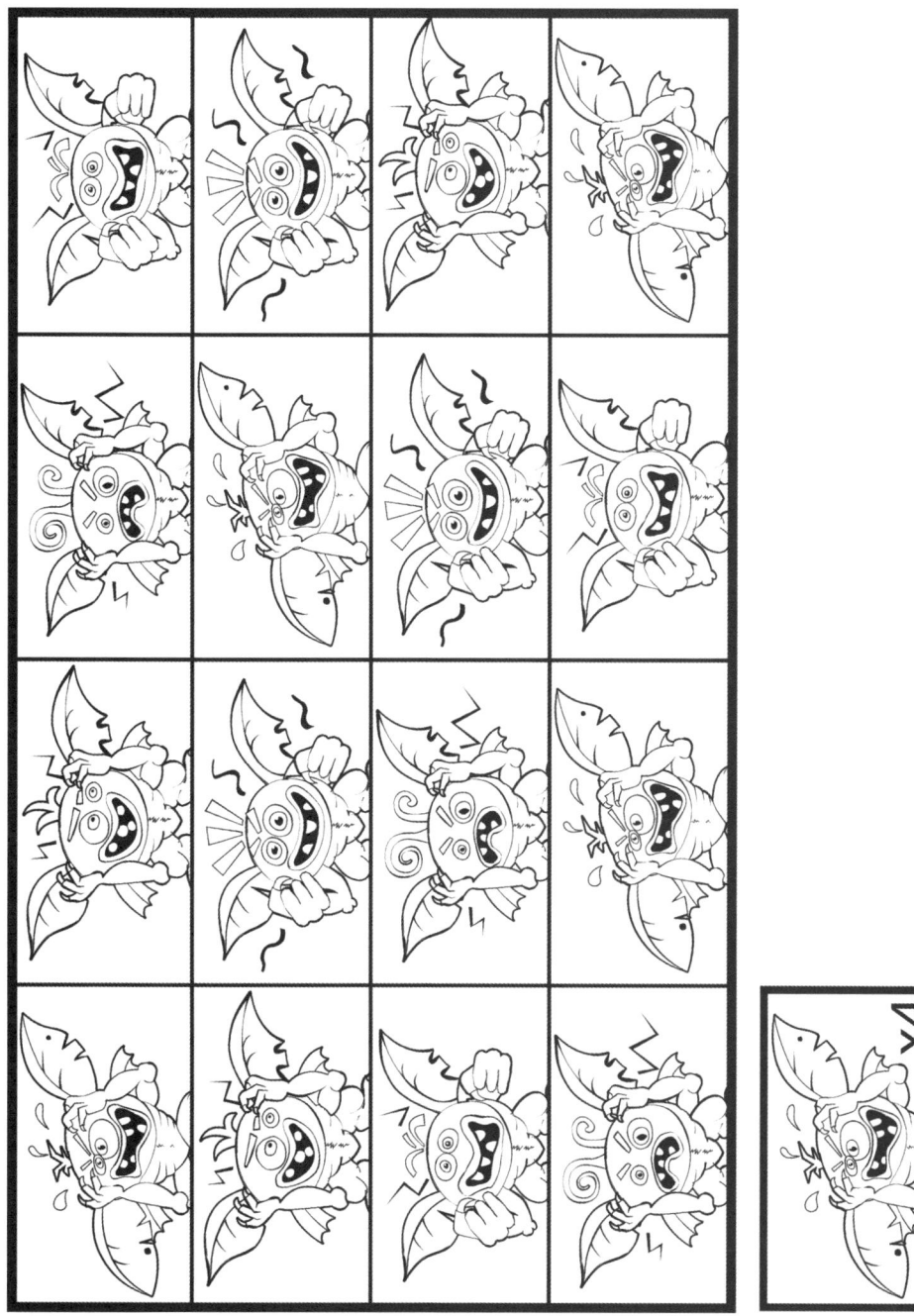

Word Jigsaw

The letter tiles below contain the following important message:

THE BIGGER YOUR ANXIETY GREMLIN THE MORE ANXIOUS YOU ARE.

But the Anxiety Gremlin has jumbled up the tiles! See if you can put them back in the correct order to spell out the message! If it makes it easier, photocopy this page and cut out the tiles and put them back together like a jigsaw. Or you can draw them in the correct order at the bottom of this page.

THE	ER Y	YOU
BIGG	ANXI	GREM
OUR	LIN	THE
MORE	ETY	ARE
ANXI	OUS	

Copyright © Kate Collins-Donnelly 2014

7
Our Anxious Bodies

Step 6 in your mission to starve your Anxiety Gremlin is to learn about the physical feelings of anxiety and how they feed your Anxiety Gremlin.

Physical Feelings

When you get anxious you will have physical feelings of anxiety in your body. Complete the puzzles below to learn about different types of anxious physical feelings.

I SPY SCRAMBLE!

Below are pictures of some different physical feelings that we can have when we get anxious and labels describing them. But the Anxiety Gremlin has been naughty again and scrambled up the letters in each label.

1. See if you can unscramble the letters.
2. See how many physical feelings you can spy that begin with the letter 'S'.

I've unscrambled two of the labels for you to start you off.

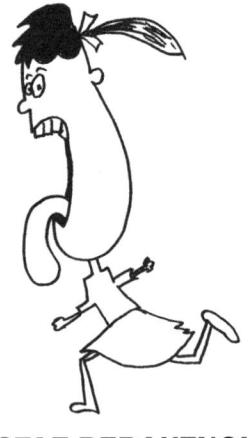

STAF BERAHTNGI

Answer: FAST BREATHING

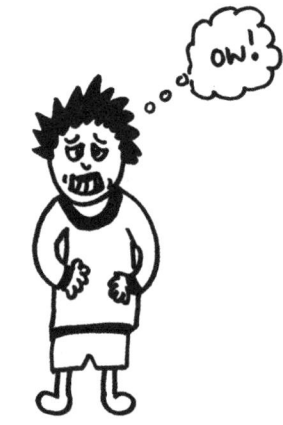

ACEH STOACHM

Answer: STOMACH ACHE

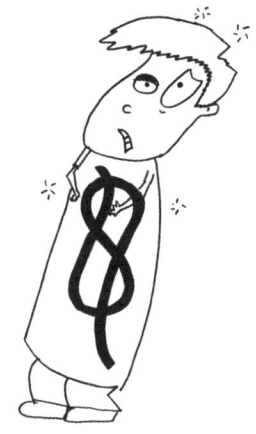

KNTO NI STOACHM

Answer:
_ _ _ _ _ _ _
_ _ _ _ _ _ _

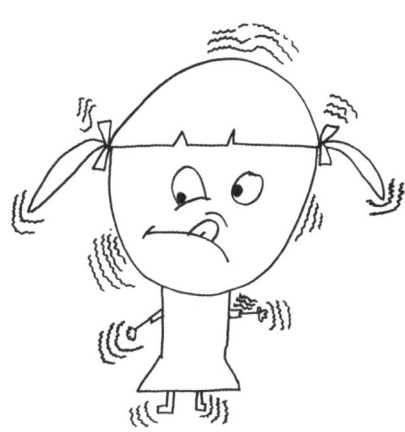

SHKIANG

Answer:
_ _ _ _ _ _ _

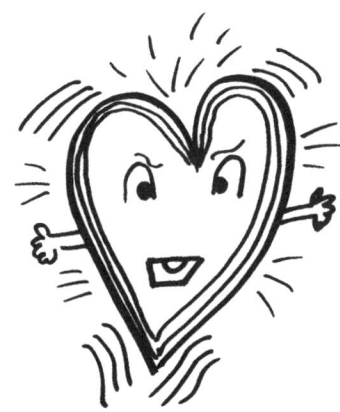

STAF HEATR BETA

Answer:
_ _ _ _
_ _ _ _ _
_ _ _ _

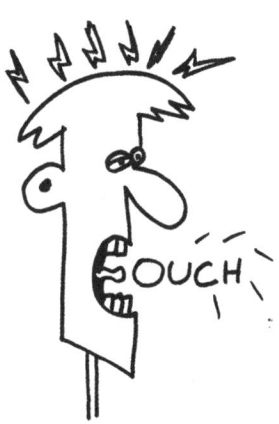

HEAACHED

Answer:
_ _ _ _ _ _ _ _

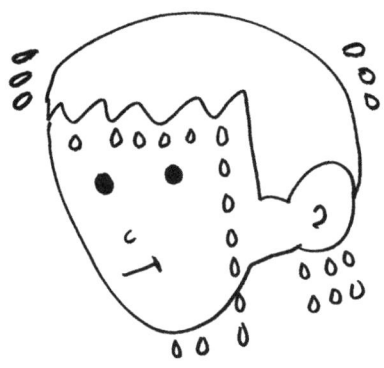

WEATNIGS

Answer:
_ _ _ _ _ _ _ _

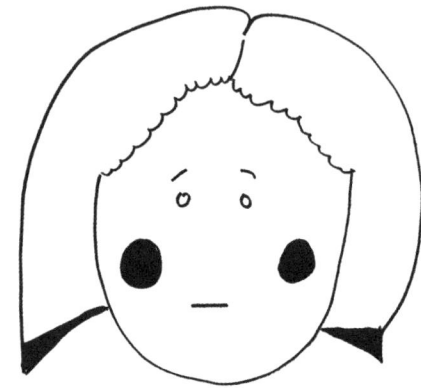

DER FAEC

Answer:
_ _ _   _ _ _ _

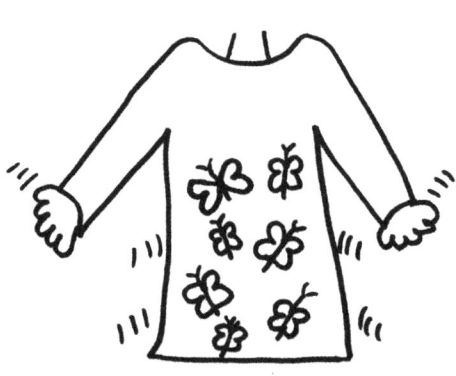

BUTTFLIEERS NI STOACHM

Answer:
_ _ _ _ _ _ _ _ _ _ _
_ _   _ _ _ _ _ _

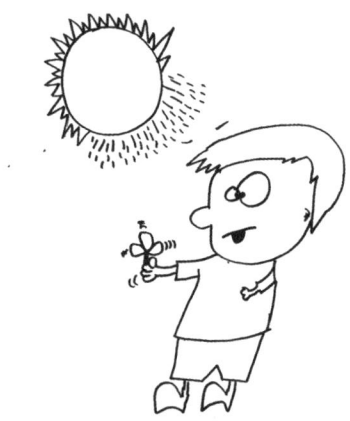

TOH

Answer:
_ _ _

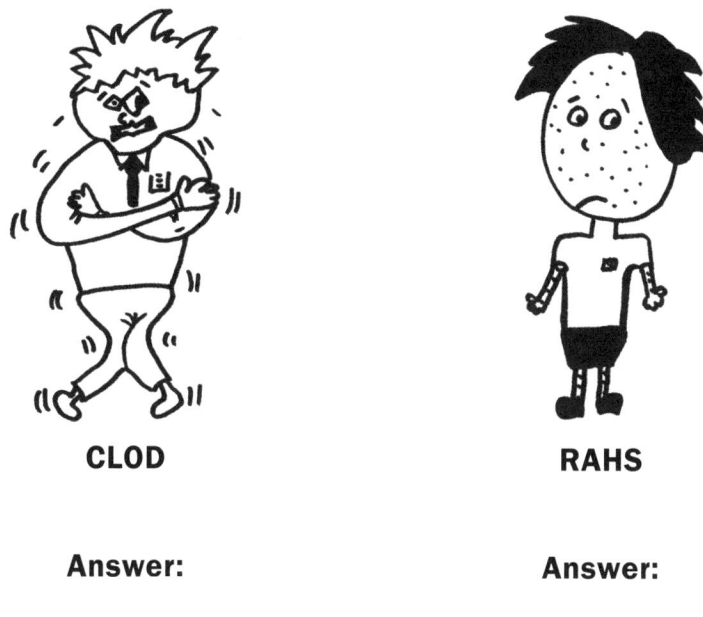

CLOD

Answer:
— — — —

RAHS

Answer:
— — — —

A Physical Match

On the next page are more pictures of physical symptoms that people can sometimes experience when they get anxious. But the Anxiety Gremlin has been naughty again. This time he has put the wrong label on each picture. See if you can match up the right picture with the right label by drawing a line between them.

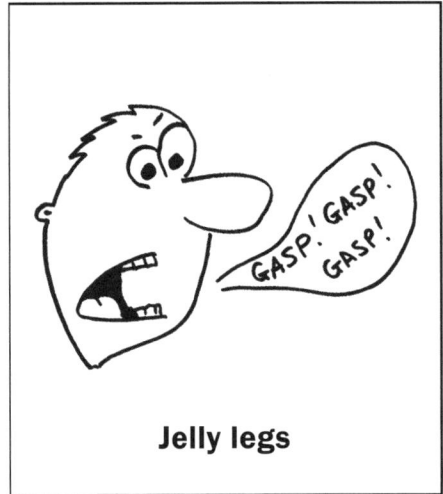
Jelly legs

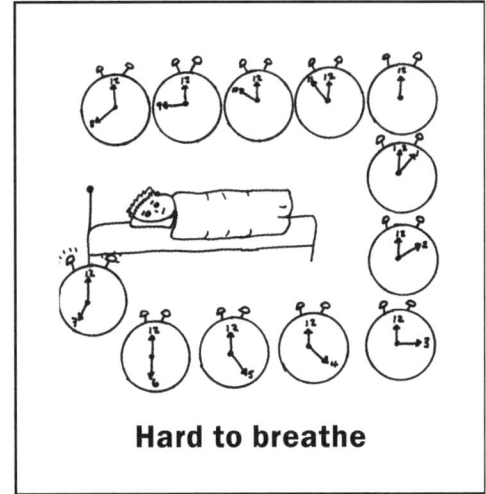
Hard to breathe

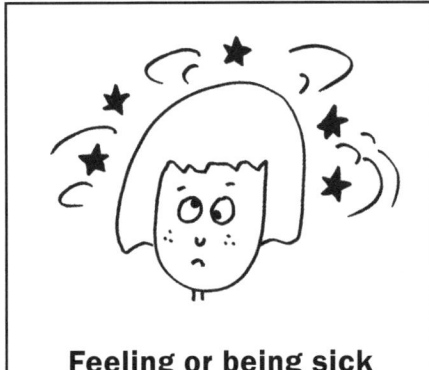
Feeling or being sick

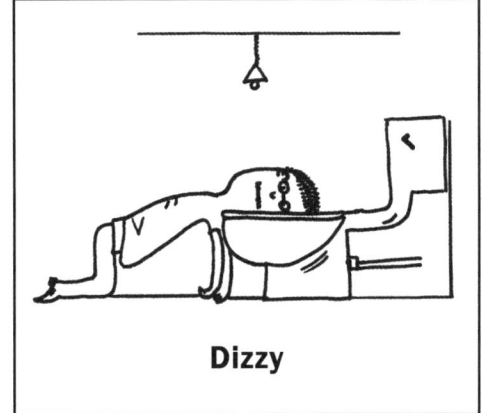
Dizzy

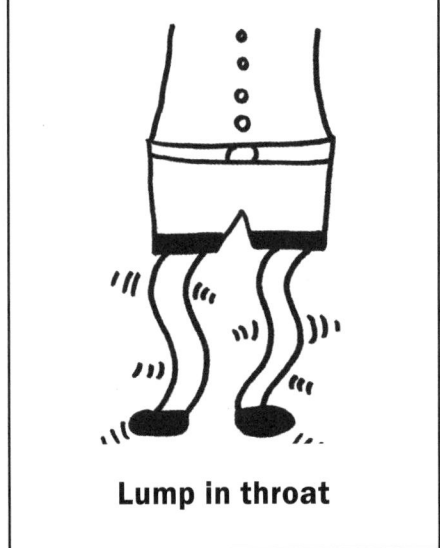
Lump in throat

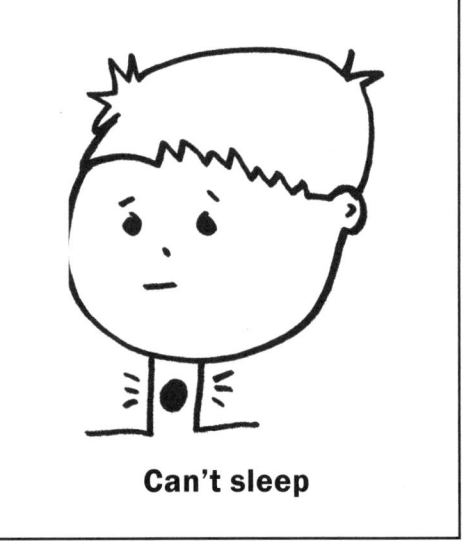
Can't sleep

Our Anxious Bodies   95

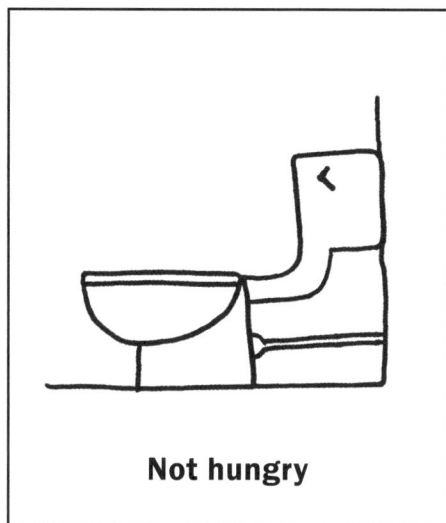
Not hungry

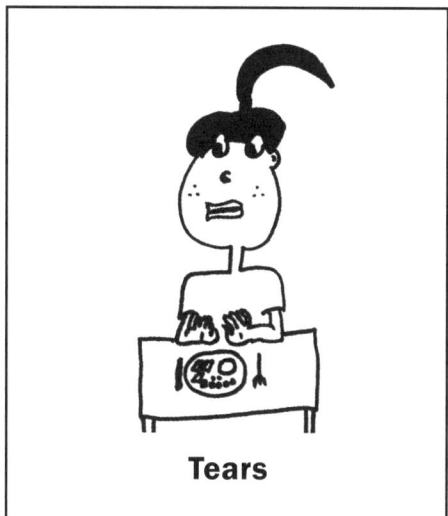
Tears

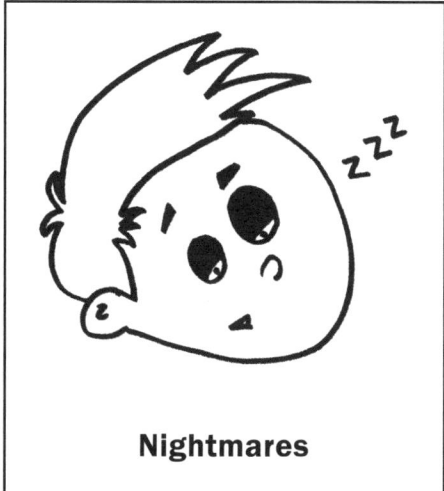
Nightmares

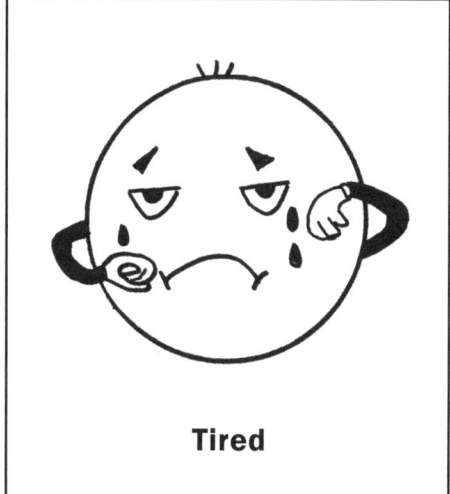
Tired

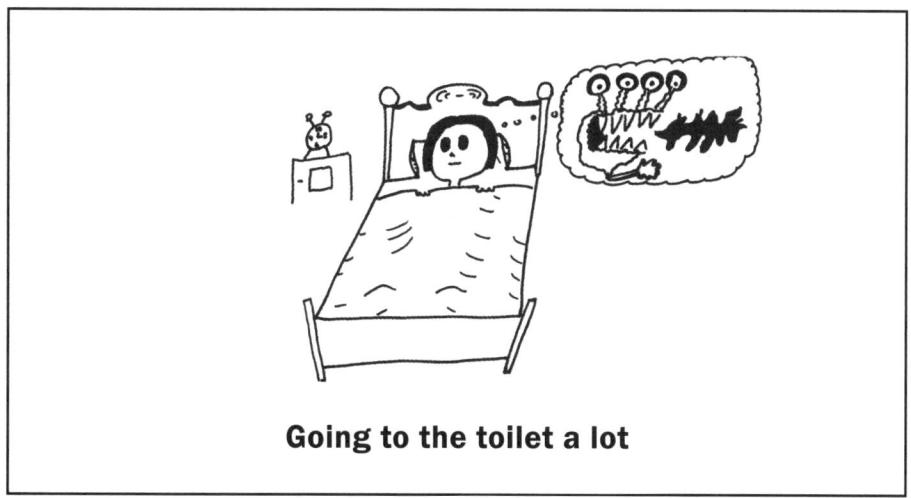
Going to the toilet a lot

Your Anxious Body

Below are the same physical feelings pictures. Circle any that you experience when you get anxious.

When I'm anxious I have...

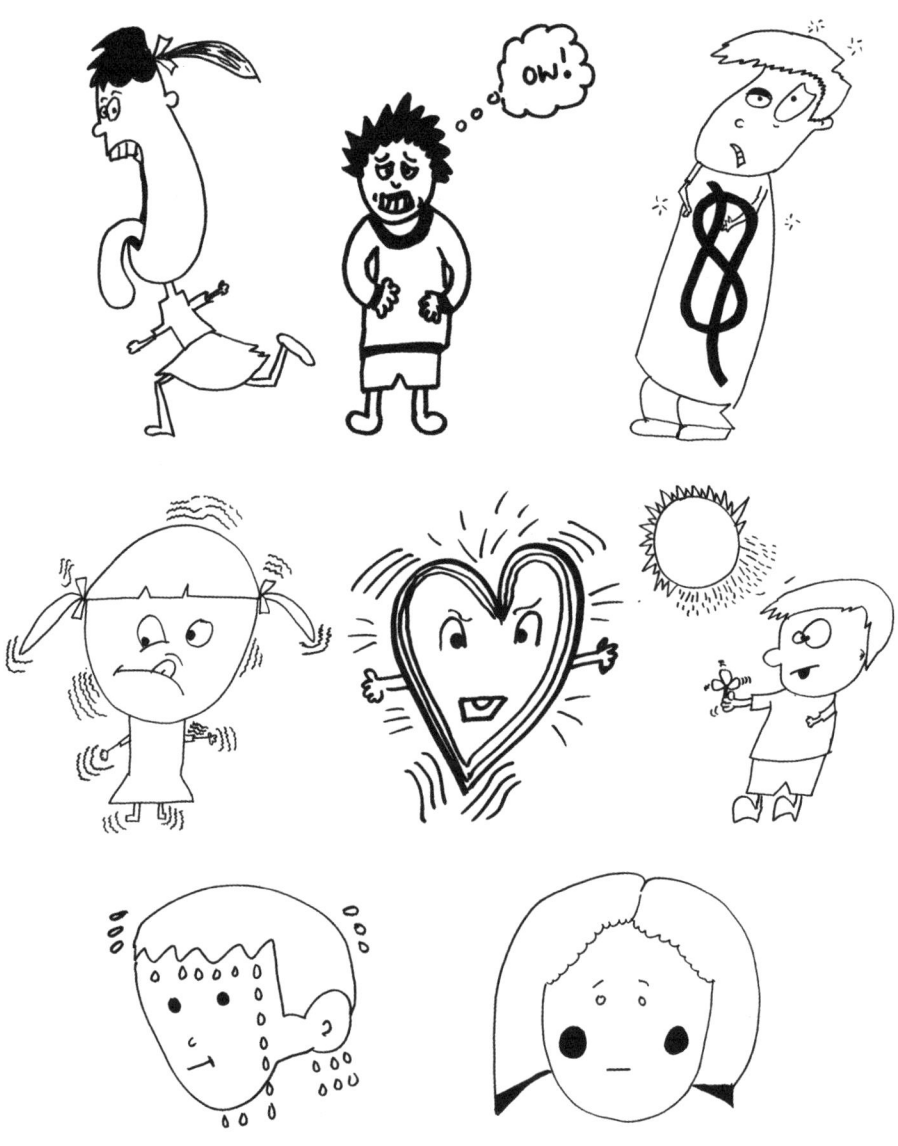

Our Anxious Bodies 97

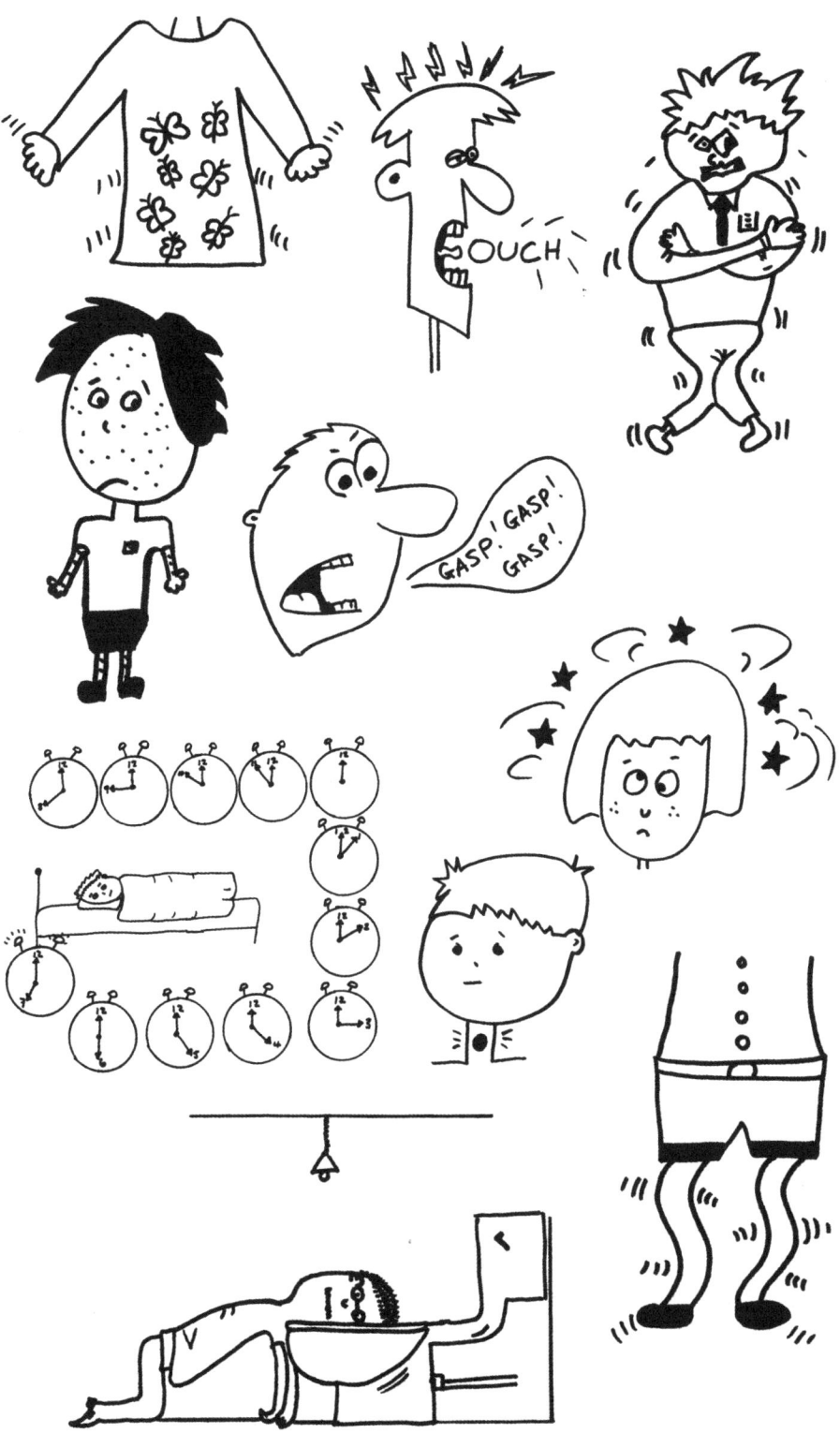

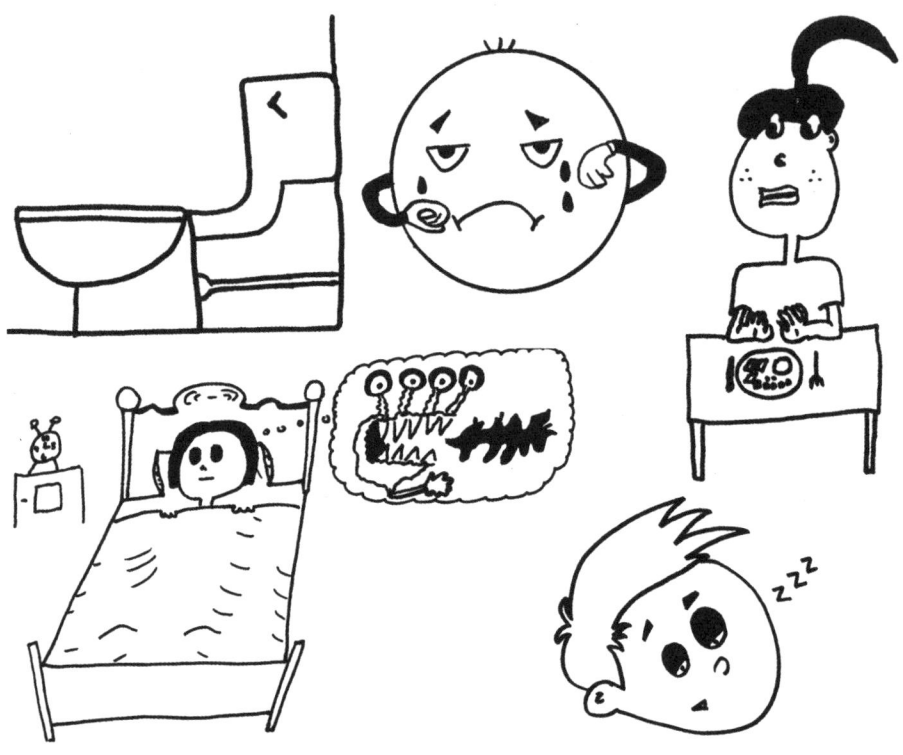

What Are Panic Attacks?

Sometimes when people are anxious they can have what is called a panic attack. A panic attack is when a person has a strong burst of one or more of the physical feelings that you have learnt about but just for a very short period of time. The most common physical feelings involved in a panic attack are:

- difficulty breathing
- fast breathing
- fast heart beat
- dizziness
- jelly legs
- shaking
- hot
- cold
- sweating
- feeling sick.

Often when people experience a panic attack, they believe it will cause them serious harm, for example that they will stop breathing. But panic attacks alone are not dangerous. They are very unpleasant and uncomfortable, but they only last for a short time.

How Physical Feelings Feed Your Anxiety Gremlin

The more anxious physical feelings you have, the more you feed your Anxiety Gremlin! And the bigger he continues to get! And the bigger he gets, the more anxious you get.

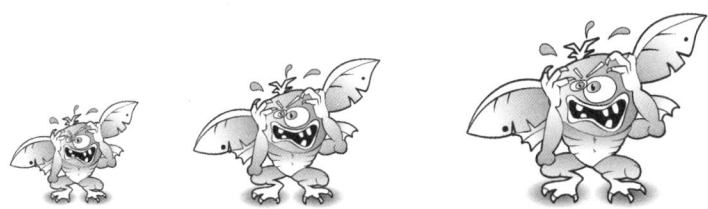

Well done for completing Step 6 in starving your Anxiety Gremlin. You are making excellent progress! Colour in your sixth **Starving the Anxiety Gremlin Star** as your reward.

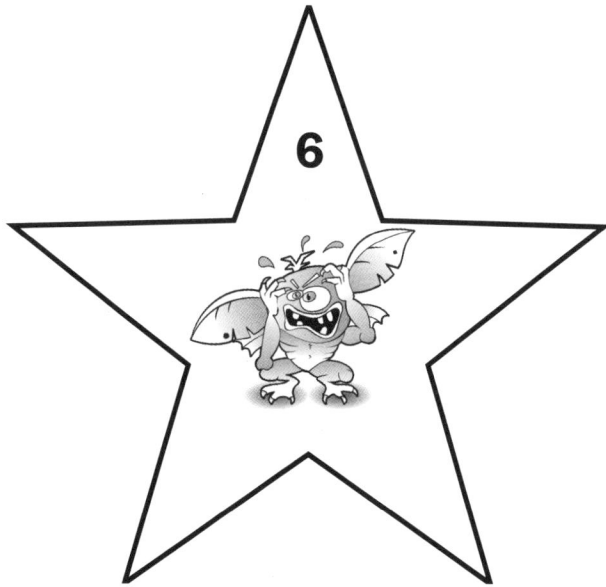

Now complete one or both of the following **Just for Fun Puzzles** as a reward for being such a hard worker! Enjoy!

The Anxiety Gremlin Goes Line Dancing!

One of the lines below leads to the Anxiety Gremlin. Have a guess which one you think it is, then trace them with your finger to find out if you are correct!

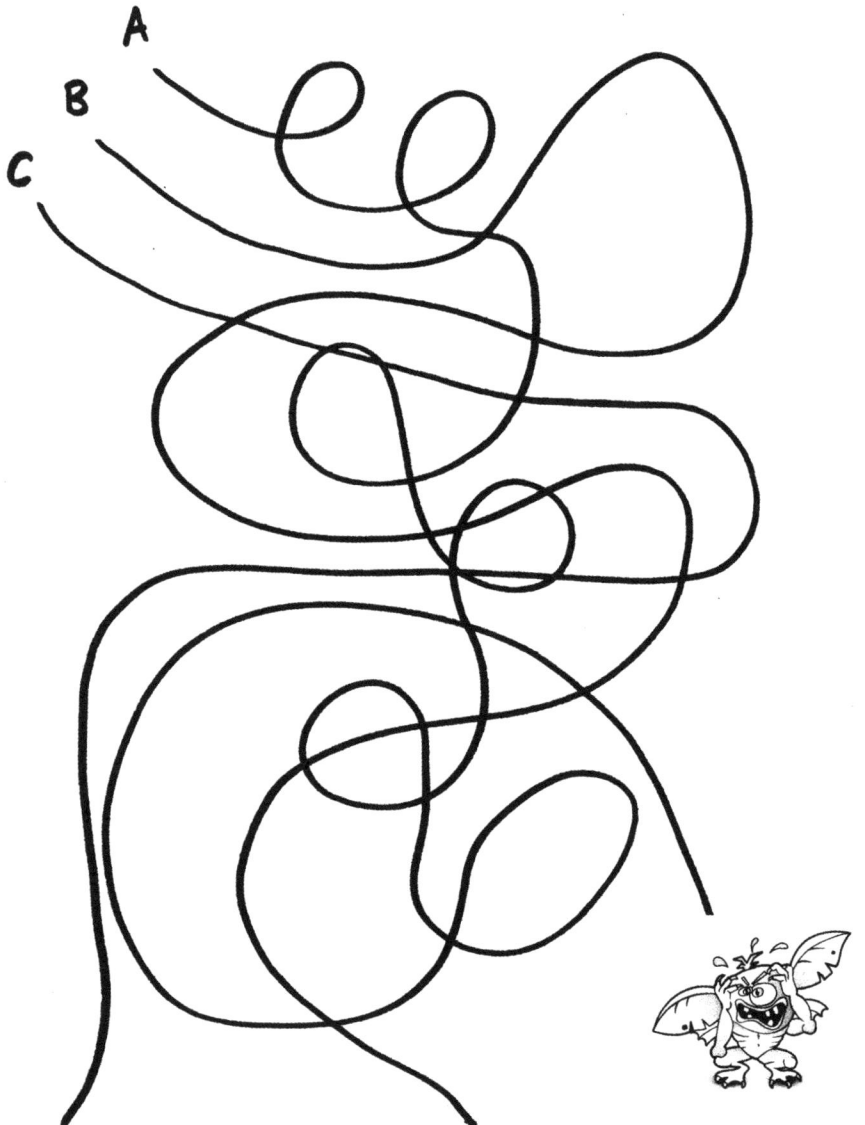

Draw the Anxiety Gremlin!

Draw the Anxiety Gremlin in the grid below square by square.

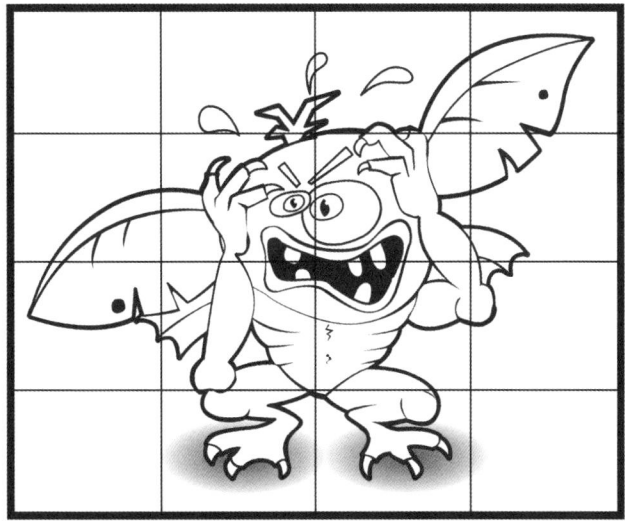

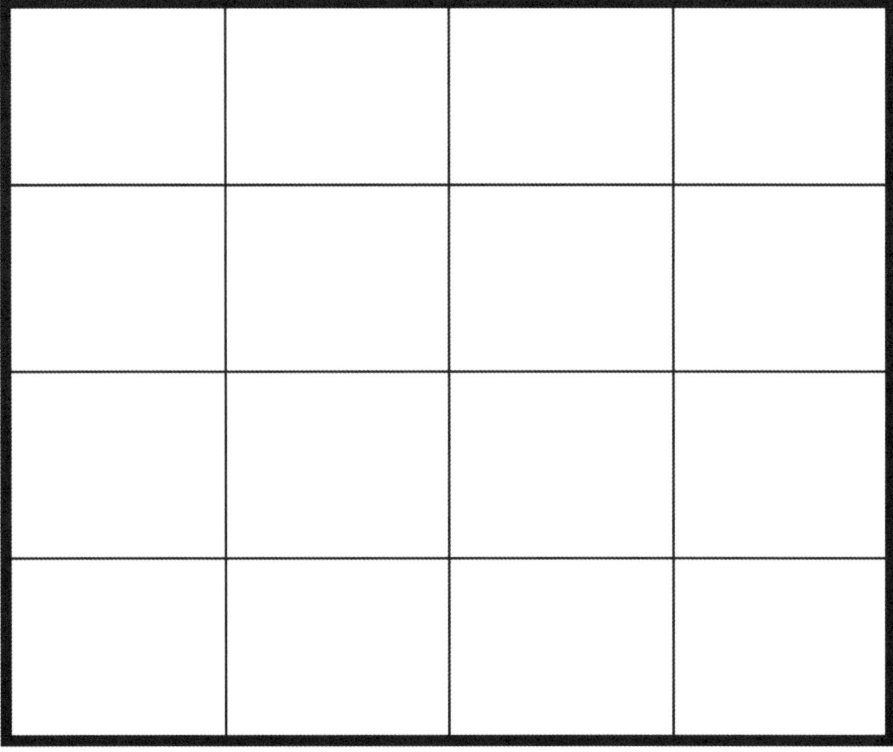

8
Our Anxious Behaviours

Step 7 in your mission to starve your Anxiety Gremlin is to learn about anxious behaviours that aren't good for you.

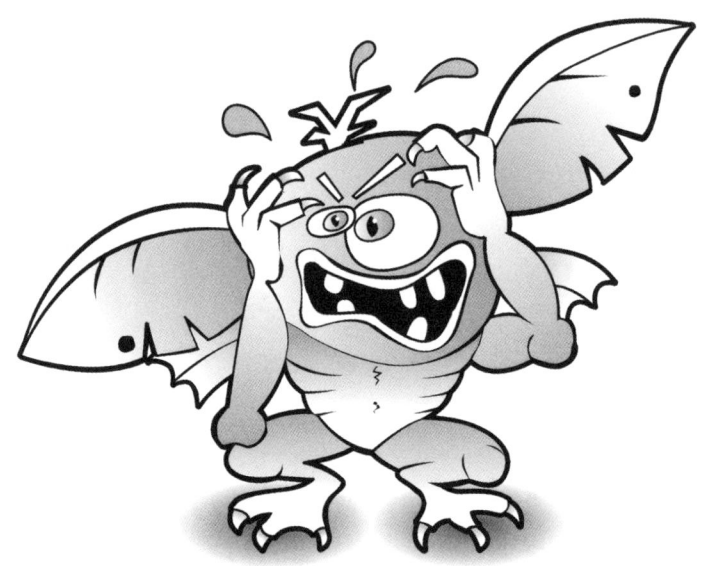

Anxious Behaviours

When we get anxious we can act in a number of different ways. Some of these behaviours aren't good for us. Here's how some of the children you met in Chapter 5 behave when they get anxious. These behaviours aren't good for them!

> Sally is six years old and she is afraid of spiders. She worries everywhere she goes in case she sees a spider. If she sees a spider she runs away!
>
> **Sally escapes!**

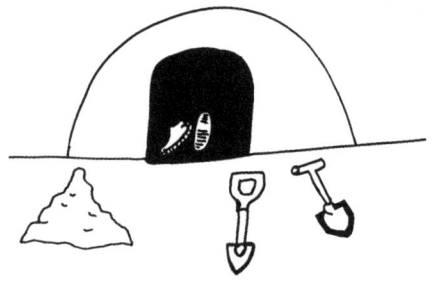

Max is seven years old and he worries all the time about something bad happening to his parents when he is not with them. Max tries to stay close to his parents all of the time and phones to check on them over and over again when he's not with them.

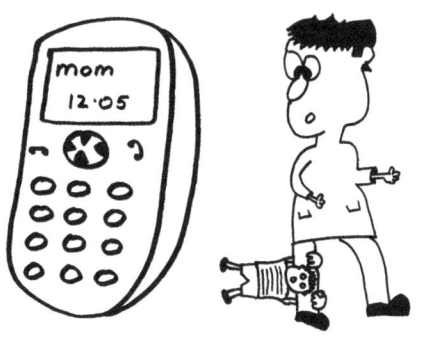

Max stays close to his parents and checks on them!

Fiona is seven years old. She once vomited during a school assembly as she had a tummy bug. She now worries every week about whether she will vomit again during assembly. She is always begging her mum to tell her that she won't be sick.

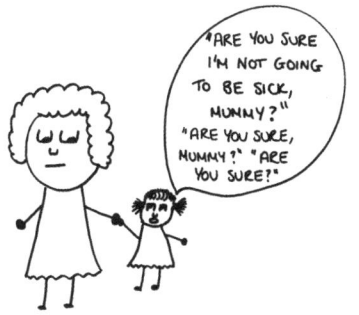

Fiona always asks her mum if everything will be OK!

Tim is eight years old and he is afraid of the dark. He avoids sleeping alone.

Tim avoids!

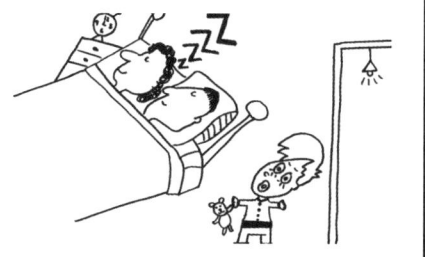

David is seven years old and he worries all the time that the other children at school don't like him and will laugh at him. He talks to his dad at home, but refuses to speak to anyone at school, including the children and his teacher.

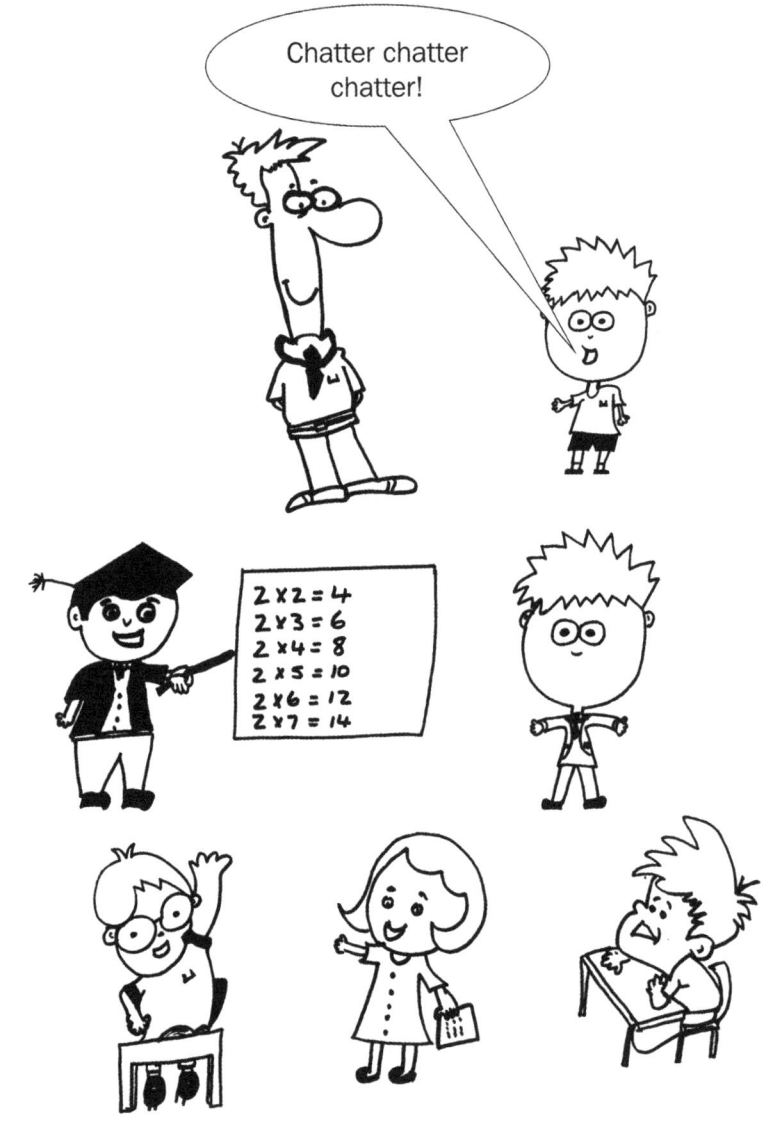

David refuses to talk at school!

Melissa is five years old and she is afraid of thunderstorms. She worries about going to school every day in case there is a thunderstorm when she is there. So Melissa pretends to be sick a lot to avoid going to school.

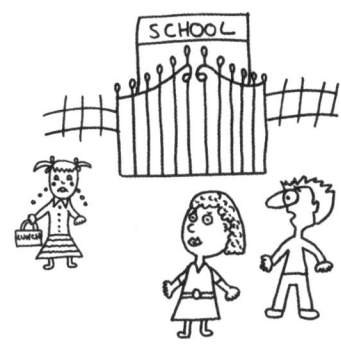

Melissa avoids!

Carla is nine years old and she worries all the time about going to the toilet in other people's houses. So Carla avoids going to parties and sleepovers at her friends' houses.

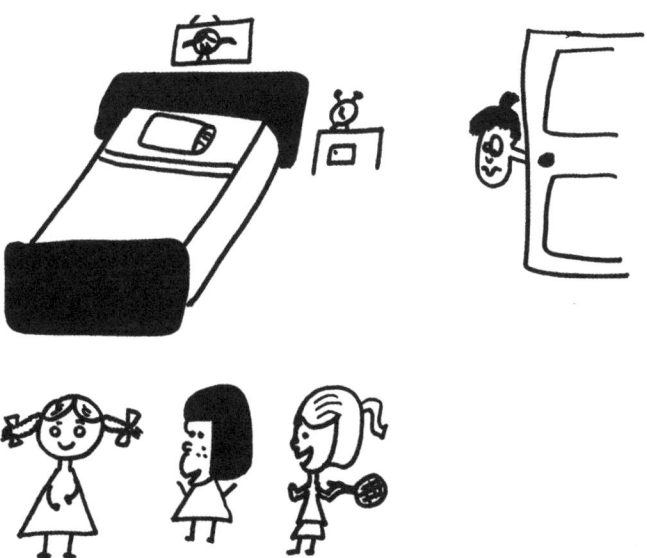

Carla avoids!

Neela is eight years old and she is afraid of dogs. She avoids getting too close to dogs. She will only go to the park with her friends if she has her favourite teddy with her for comfort as she knows there are normally dogs in the park.

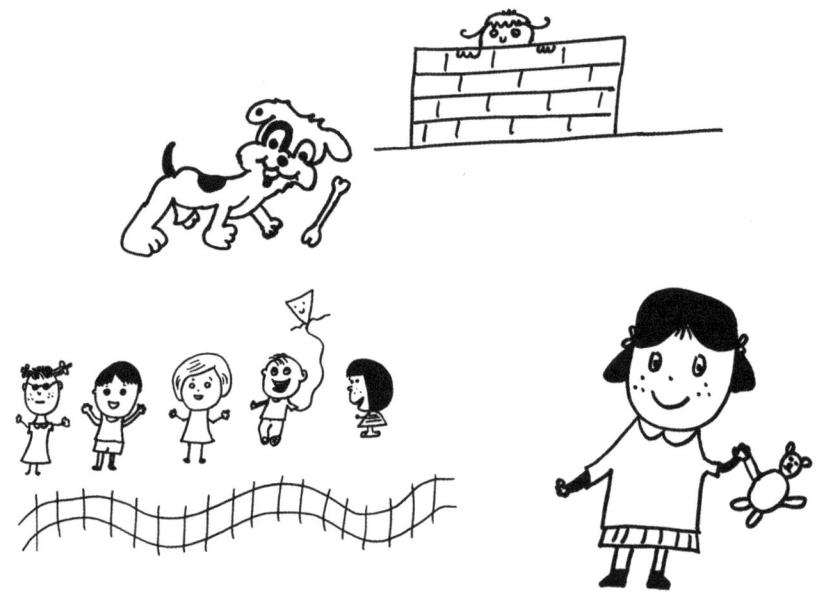

Neela avoids and uses her teddy as a comfort!

Grace is six years old and she is afraid of leaving the house so she stays at home all of the time.

Grace stays inside the house!

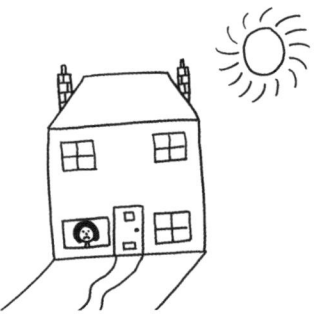

Our Anxious Behaviours   109

Freddie is eight years old and he worries that bad things will happen if he doesn't put his pencils back in a certain order in his pencil case and if his teddies aren't in a certain order in his room. He feels that he has to check his pencil case at least ten times a day and he shouts at his mum if she doesn't put his teddies back in the correct order when she makes his bed.

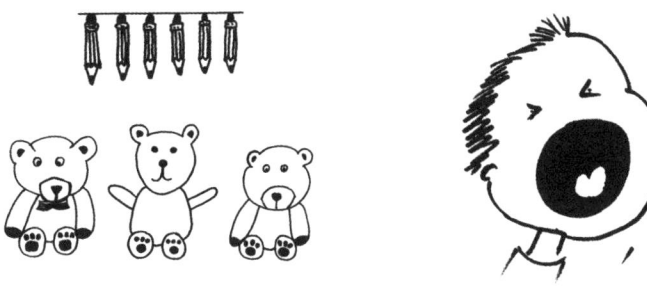

Freddie checks and organises things and shouts!

Helen is nine years old and she worries all the time about catching germs and getting poorly. Helen hides from other people and washes her hands over and over again!

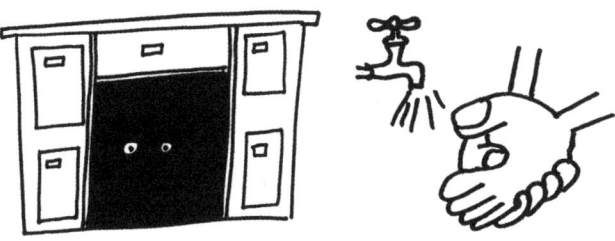

Helen hides and washes her hands a lot!

Your Anxious Behaviours

Below are the same anxious behaviours pictures. Circle any that you do when you get anxious.

When I'm anxious I...

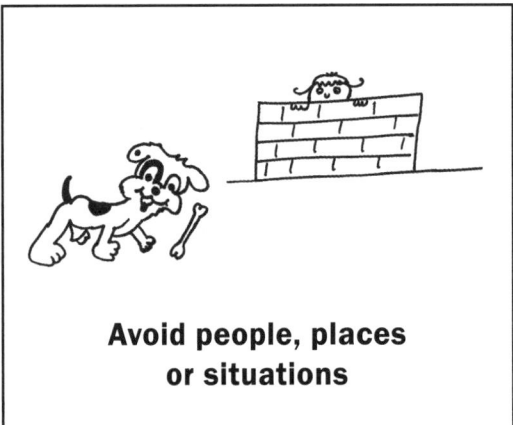

Avoid people, places or situations

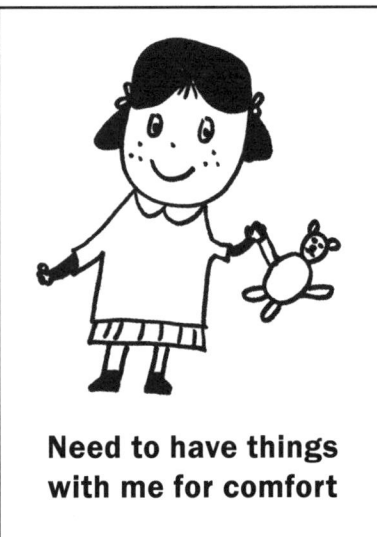

Need to have things with me for comfort

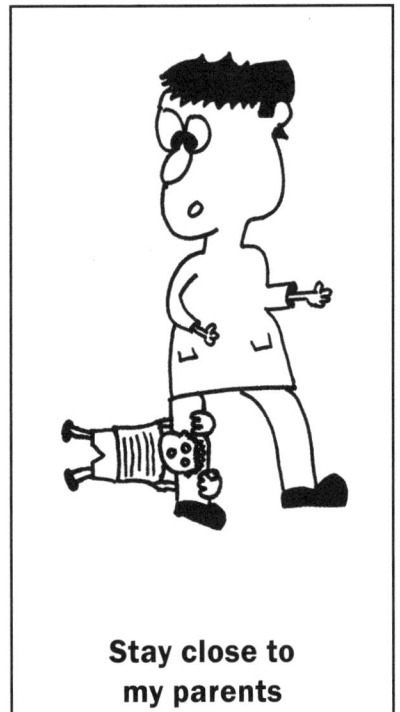

Stay close to my parents

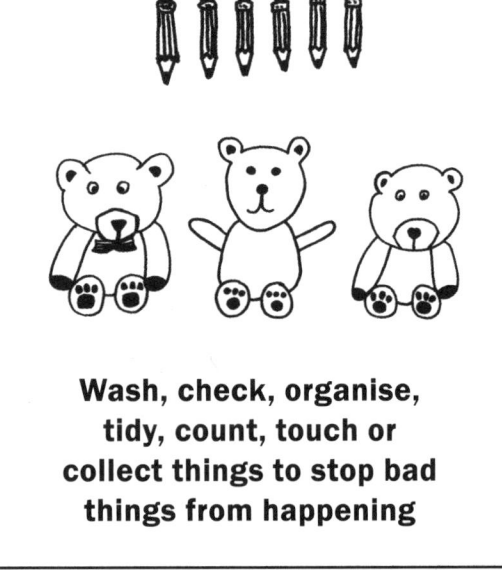

Wash, check, organise, tidy, count, touch or collect things to stop bad things from happening

Our Anxious Behaviours

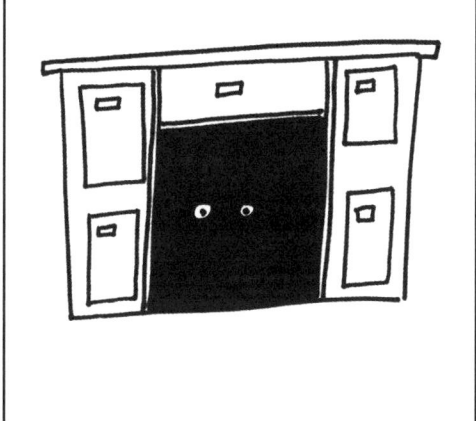

Hide from people, places or situations

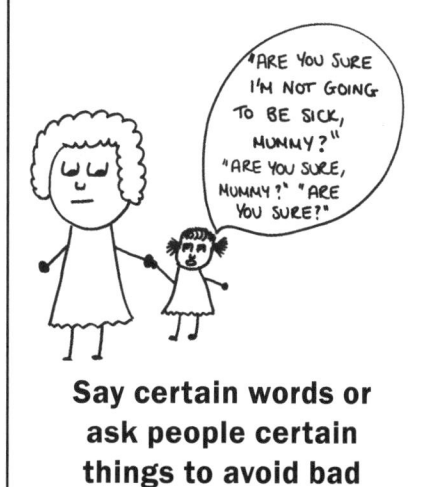

Say certain words or ask people certain things to avoid bad things happening

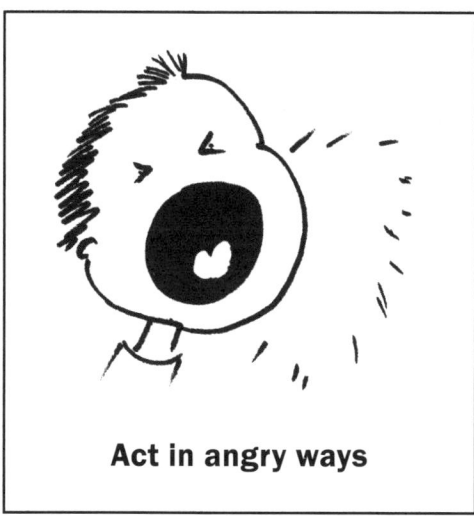

Act in angry ways

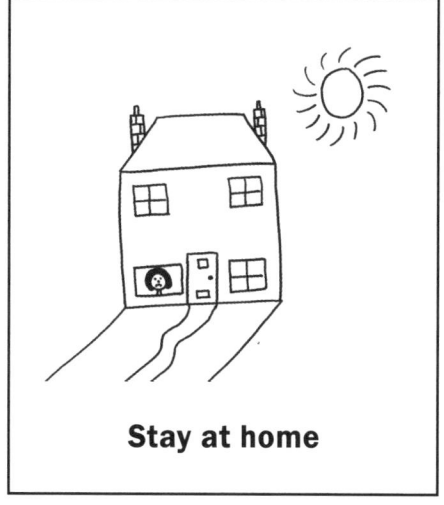

Stay at home

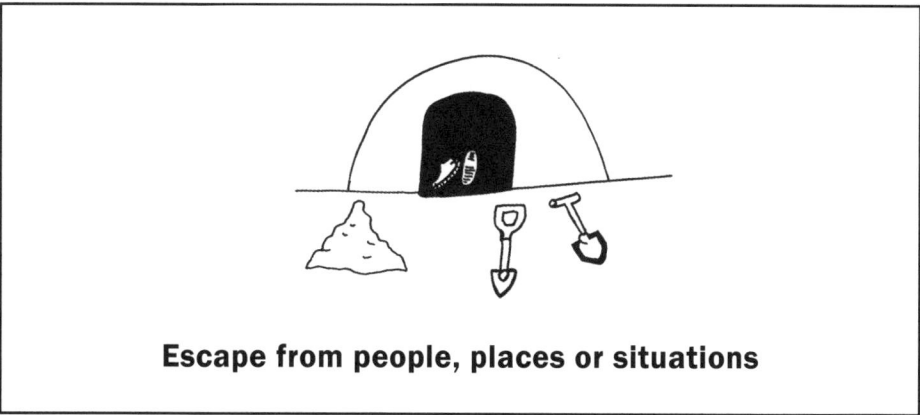

Escape from people, places or situations

How Anxious Behaviours Feed Your Anxiety Gremlin

If you act in ways that aren't good for you when you're anxious, you feed your Anxiety Gremlin. The more you feed him by acting in these ways, the bigger he gets and the more likely it is that you will get anxious more often!

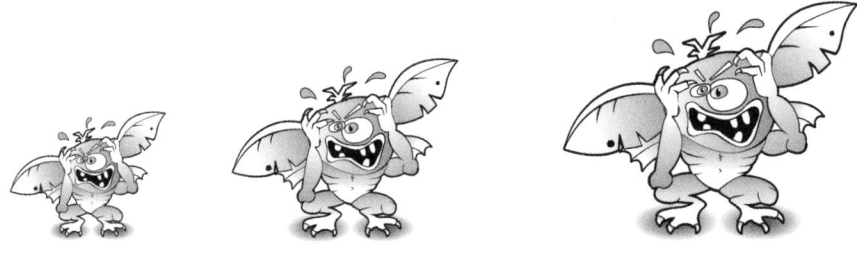

How Often Do You Get Anxious?

QUESTION: How often do you feel anxious? Circle your answer.

Most of the time   Often   Sometimes

Rarely   Never

The more you get anxious, the more you feed your Anxiety Gremlin and he continues to grow and grow.

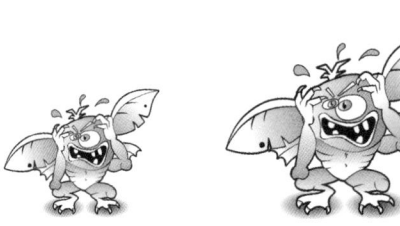 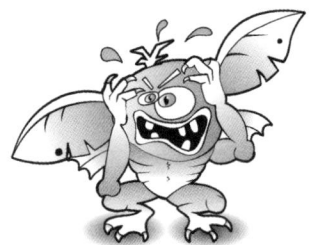

The results are lots of bad effects for you.

Congratulate yourself on completing Step 7 in starving your Anxiety Gremlin and colour in your seventh **Starving the Anxiety Gremlin Star** as your reward.

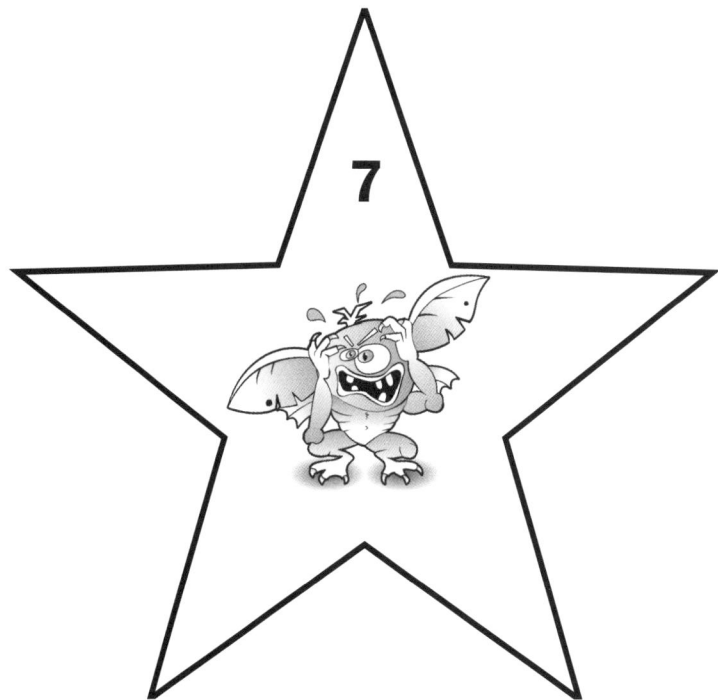

Now complete one or both of the following **Just for Fun Puzzles** as a reward for all your amazing learning so far! Enjoy!

Spot the Difference

Below are two pictures. Although they might look identical at first glance, they aren't! See if you can spot the eight differences between the two pictures. Mark the differences on the bottom picture. Have fun!

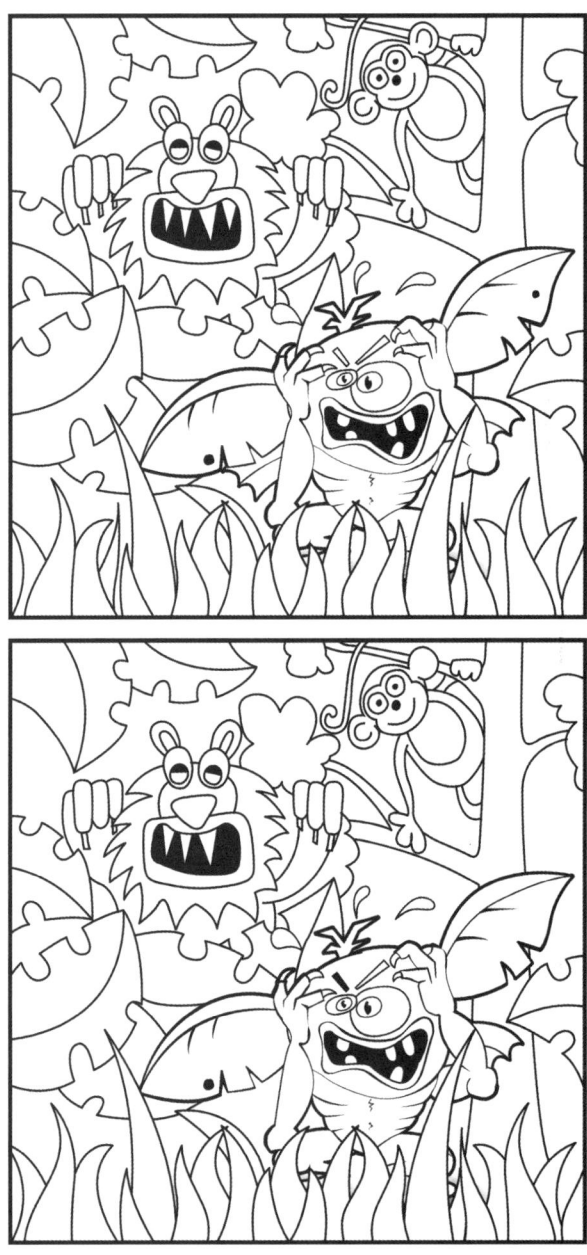

Find the Missing Letters

I have written a sentence below but the Anxiety Gremlin has stolen a letter from each word in the sentence! There are replacement letters in tiles at the bottom of the page. Put the right letter in the right place to complete the sentence.

YO___R ANXIE___Y GRE___LIN
W___LL ___ET BIGG___R I___
___OU A___OID THIN___S
W___EN Y___U A___E
___NXIOUS.

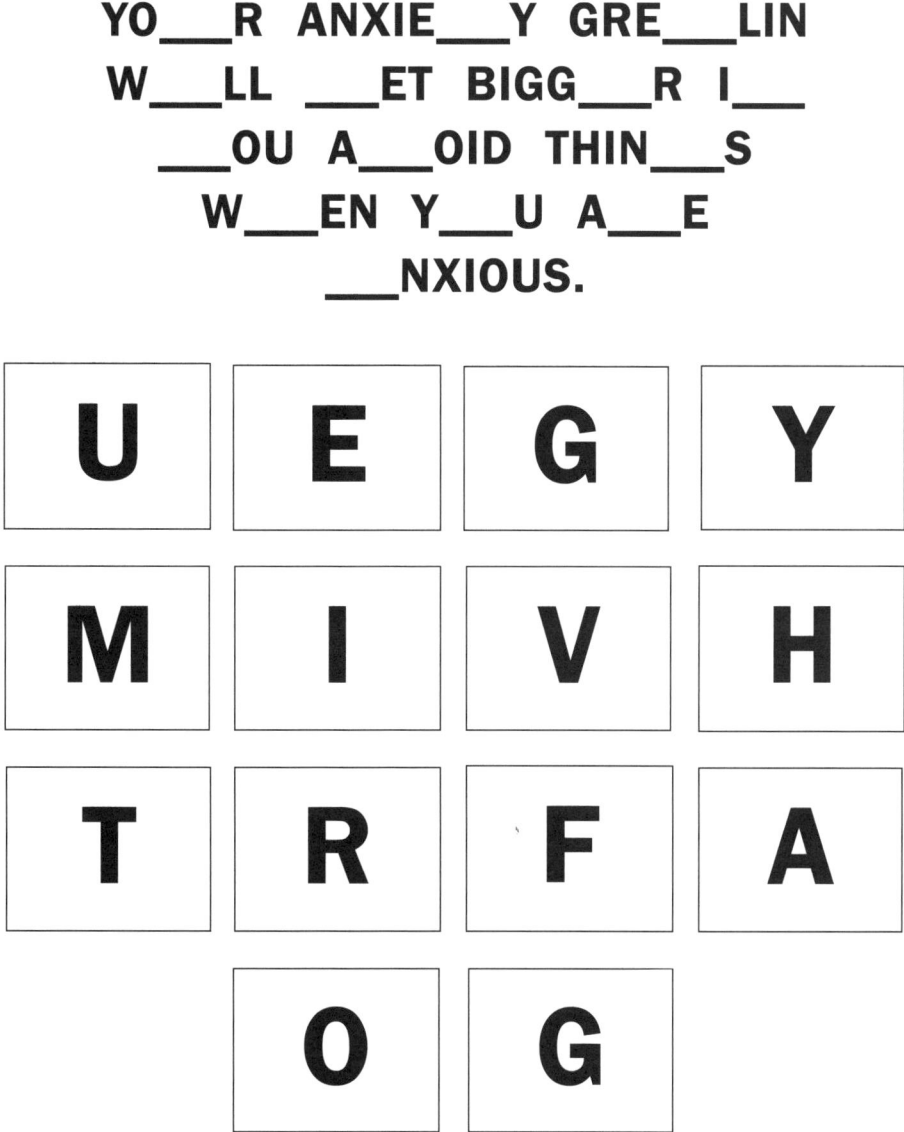

9
The Effects Anxiety Can Have

Step 8 in your mission to starve your Anxiety Gremlin is learning about the bad effects that feeling anxious can have on you. Let's look at what some of these can be through a number of activities!

What Happens Next?

Below is a story about a six-year-old boy called Danny. But it's not finished. I would like you to read the story so far and then write or draw its ending! Make sure your ending shows the effects that Danny's anxiety has on him.

Who Wants to Be Beside the Seaside?

Danny's class at St Michael's School are going on a school trip to the seaside. Danny loves the sea and really wants to go on the school trip, but he is worried about going.

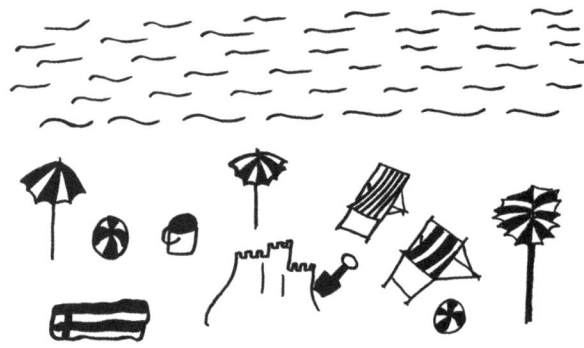

When Danny was five years old, he went on holiday with his mum and dad to stay in a holiday park in a beautiful forest. It took them a long time to travel to the forest by car and on the way, Danny got travel sick. Danny always gets worried about going on journeys now as he is afraid he will get travel sick again, even though he has been on many long journeys since and hasn't been travel sick during any of them.

The Effects Anxiety Can Have

Danny worries for weeks and weeks before the school trip. He can't sleep and he has nightmares about feeling sick. By the time the day of the school trip comes, Danny is exhausted, his stomach hurts and he cannot stop shaking.

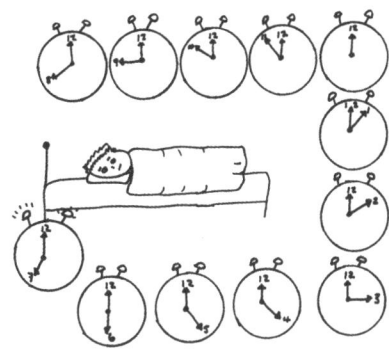

'Are you sure you want to go on the trip today, sweetie pie?' asks Danny's mum. Danny just nods. He feels like he can't speak because of the lump in his throat that his worry is causing.

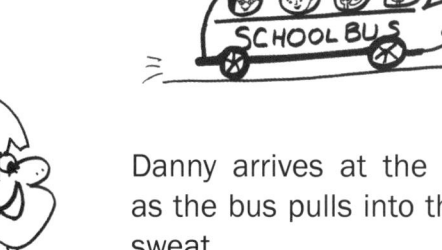

Danny arrives at the school gates and watches as the bus pulls into the school yard. He starts to sweat.

Danny's best friend, Oscar, runs past him shouting, 'Hurry up, Danny! Otherwise the best seats on the bus will be gone!'

But Danny feels like he cannot move. 'What do I do if I feel sick?' Danny asks his mum for the hundredth time that morning.

'You will be just fine, Danny,' says his mum with a reassuring smile.

Danny nods at his mum and walks slowly over to the bus. But as he puts his foot on the first step, he freezes. His heart starts to beat really fast. He starts to feel really dizzy. He feels like he will never be able to stop shaking. Danny bursts into tears and shouts, 'Mum, I can't go!'

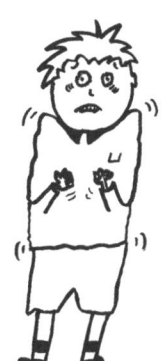

Please Continue in the Box on the Next Page!

[Blank drawing box]

Now answer the following questions about the story you have just read.

QUESTION: Did Danny see things through Anxiety Thinking Glasses? Circle your answer.

Yes   No

QUESTION: What physical feelings of anxiety did Danny have?

....

....

QUESTION: How did Danny act?

....

....

QUESTION: Which of the following did Danny do? Circle your answer.

Starve his Anxiety Gremlin   Feed his Anxiety Gremlin

The Day I Got Anxious

Now I'd like you to write your own story or draw a comic strip called 'The Day I Got Anxious'. You can use the box below or a separate piece of paper.

The Day I Got Anxious

Now answer the following questions about the day you got anxious.

QUESTION: Did you see things through Anxiety Thinking Glasses? Circle your answer.

Yes　　　　　　　　No

QUESTION: What physical feelings of anxiety did you have?

....
....

QUESTION: How did you act?

....
....

QUESTION: Which of the following did you do? Circle your answer.

Starve your Anxiety Gremlin　　　　Feed your Anxiety Gremlin

QUESTION: What effects did your anxiety have on you?

....
....
....
....

Effects of Anxiety on You

If you get anxious a lot it can have lots of bad effects on you. Here are some pictures showing you some of the effects that anxiety can have. Circle or colour in the pictures that show how your anxiety has affected you.

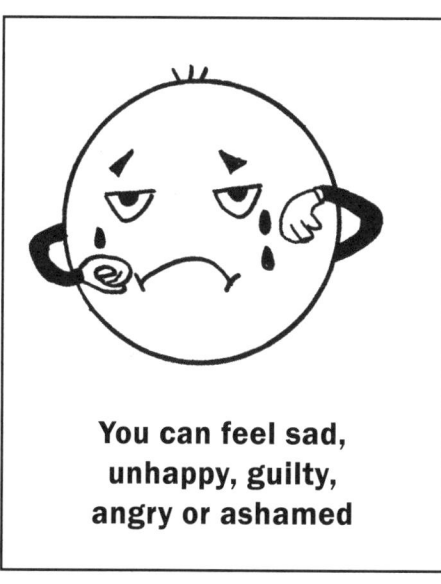

You can feel sad, unhappy, guilty, angry or ashamed

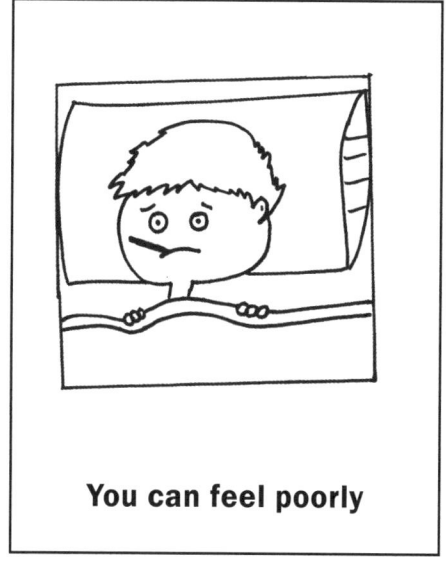

You can feel poorly

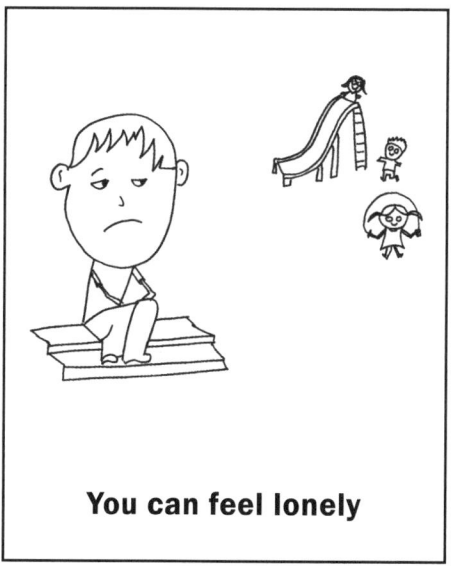

You can feel lonely

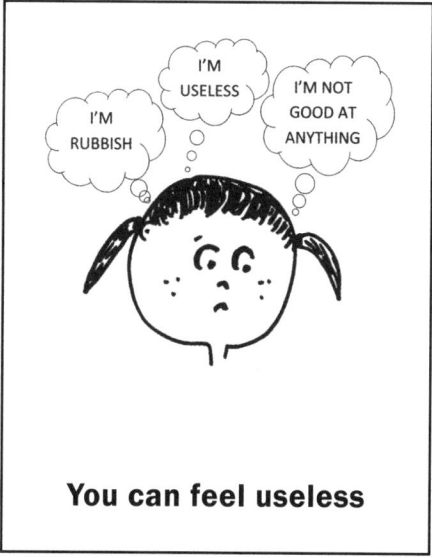

You can feel useless

You can get lower grades at school because you can't concentrate

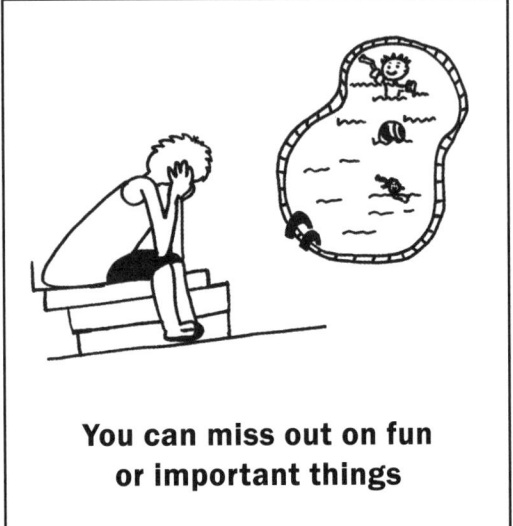

You can miss out on fun or important things

Here is something you may not have realised until now...the more of these bad effects that you experience, the harder it will be to stop feeling anxious. So you are more likely to carry on feeding your Anxiety Gremlin until he gets so big he is...

MASSIVE

HUGE

ENORMOUS

and even

The Effects Anxiety Can Have

GINORMOUS!

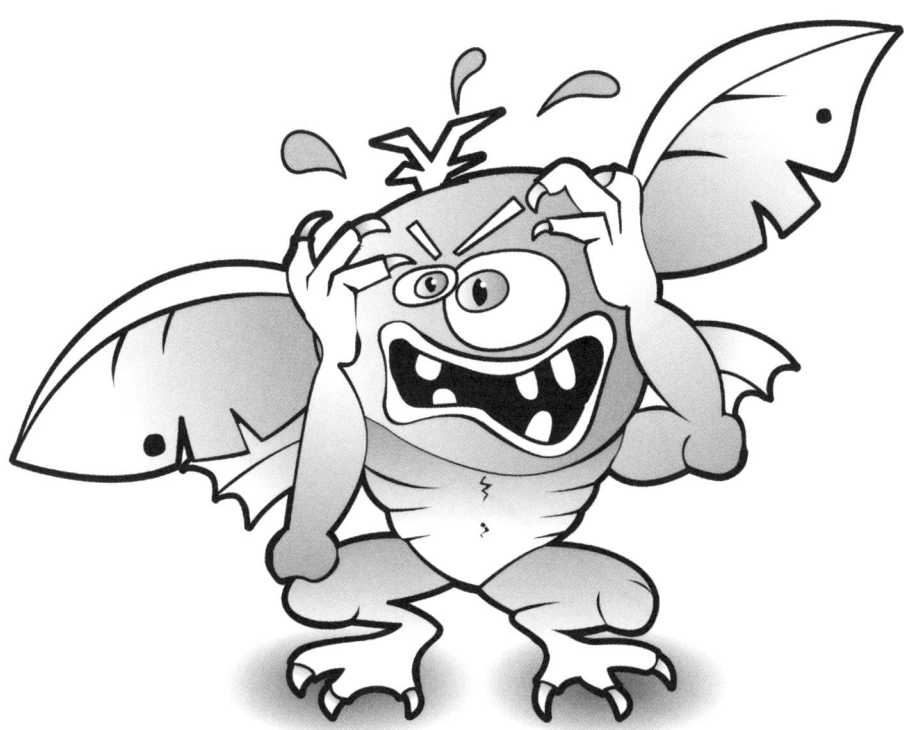

And when this happens you will feel like it is impossible to stop being anxious. It will feel like you have no control over your anxiety. But guess what? You do!

You are in control of your anxiety because you have the choice to feed or starve your Anxiety Gremlin!

Reward yourself for completing Step 8 in starving your Anxiety Gremlin by colouring in your eighth **Starving the Anxiety Gremlin Star**!

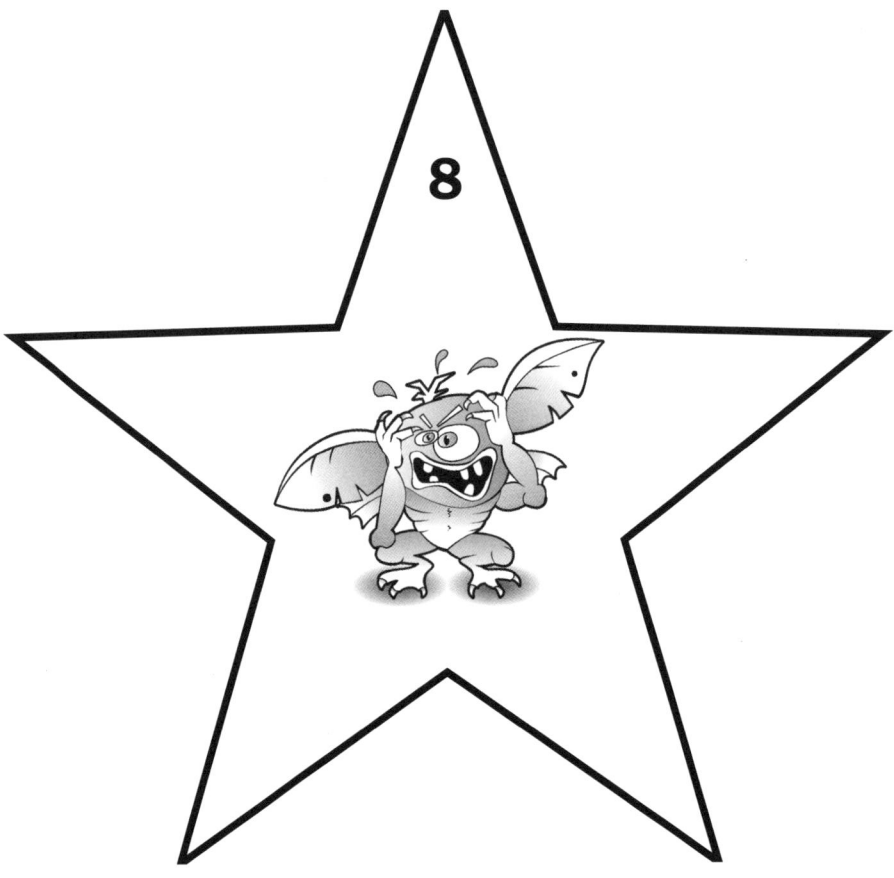

Now complete one or both of the following **Just for Fun Puzzles** as a reward for working so hard! You are doing so well!

Hidden Gremlins!

There are five Anxiety Gremlins hidden in the picture on the next page. See if you can spot all five! Mark the Gremlins on the picture.

The Effects Anxiety Can Have   127

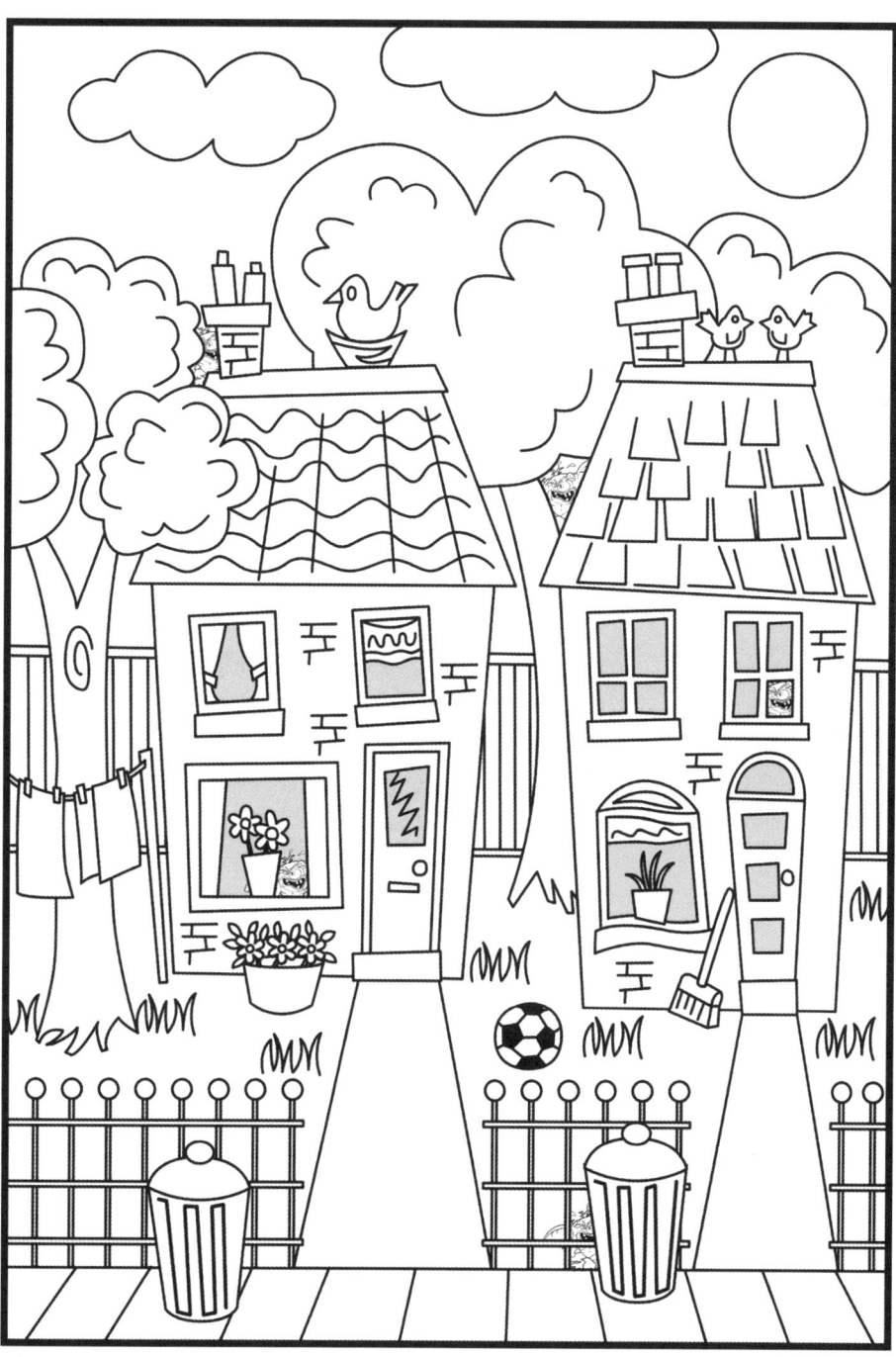

Picture Suduko

Complete the picture suduko below. You need to make sure that there is one of each of the following three pictures on each horizontal and vertical row. I have started it for you.

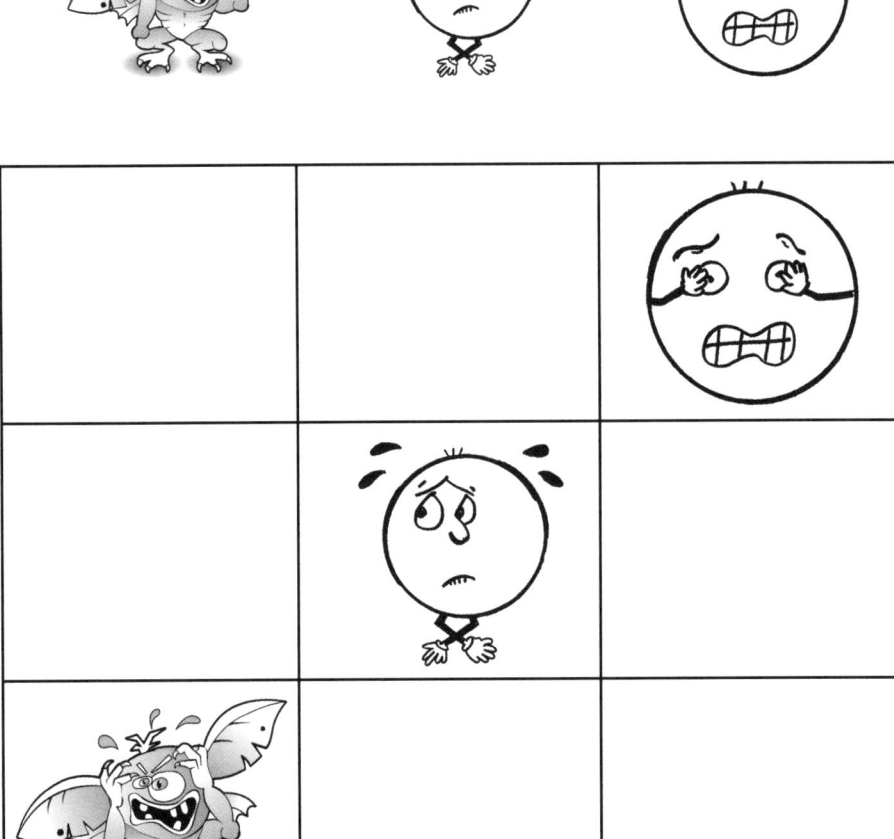

10
Starving the Anxiety Gremlin Strategies

Before you can complete your mission to starve your Anxiety Gremlin you first need to know what he looks like!

Draw Your Own Anxiety Gremlin

Think about how your Anxiety Gremlin might look and draw him in the box below or on your own piece of paper. Then give him a name! On the next page is one that was drawn by Jessie aged five years.

My Anxiety Gremlin named

....

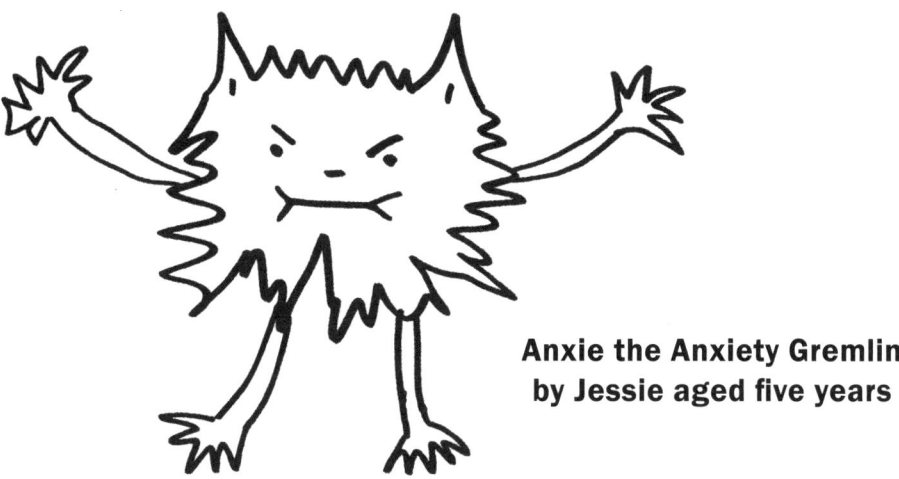

Anxie the Anxiety Gremlin by Jessie aged five years

OK, now you know what your Anxiety Gremlin looks like, let's move on to Step 9 in your mission to starve him. This involves learning how to do two things...

| Think differently | Act differently |

Think Differently

Do you remember that it is how you think about a person, animal, bird, insect, place, action or situation that causes your anxiety? Do you remember that if you think through Anxiety Thinking Glasses you are feeding your Anxiety Gremlin?

To stop this and to starve your Anxiety Gremlin you need to...

think differently!

BE A THOUGHT DETECTIVE!

When you feel yourself getting anxious, you need to try and think like a **Thought Detective** instead. This means searching for things called **facts** just like a detective searching for evidence. Facts are the things that we know are definitely true.

To search for the facts ask yourself questions such as:

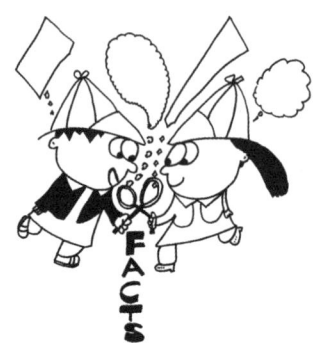

- Why am I getting anxious?
- What will the effects of my anxiety be?
- What am I thinking?
- What are the facts about the situation?
- Are my thoughts based on the facts?
- Am I thinking through Anxiety Thinking Glasses?
- Do I really need to be anxious right now?
- Is it worth getting anxious over?

Once you find the facts you can use them to think differently and starve your Anxiety Gremlin!

Once you become a Thought Detective and begin thinking differently by searching for the facts lots of things should start to happen:

- You should get anxious less and less.
- You should help to starve your Anxiety Gremlin.
- Your Anxiety Gremlin should start to shrink!

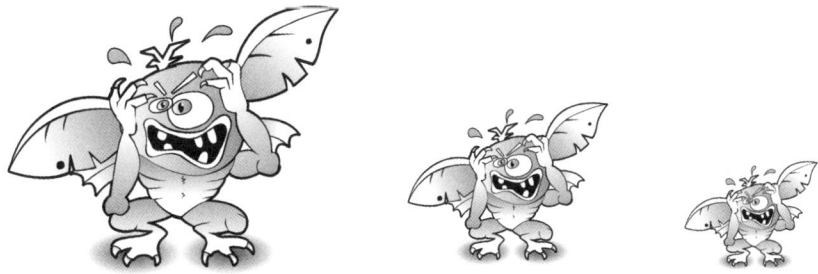

Let's practise being a Thought Detective and searching for the facts using the story below.

The School Sports Day!

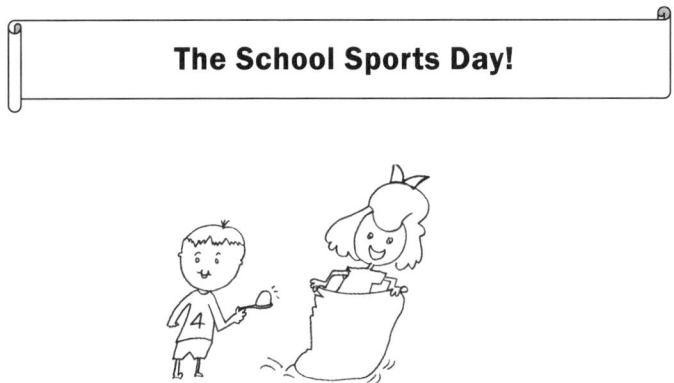

It's the day of the school sports day and all of the children are happy and excited except one! Six-year-old Sophie is very anxious!

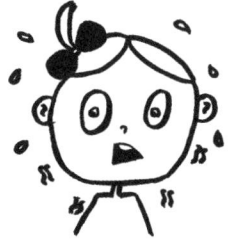

Sophie has a stutter and she gets worried whenever she has to speak or perform in front of other people. She gets worried when she has to read a book or say her times tables in front of the teacher at school. She gets worried when the teacher asks her a question in class and she has to answer it in front of all the other children. Sophie thinks that she will make a fool of herself and that people will think she is silly and laugh at her if she stutters when speaking or performing in front of them.

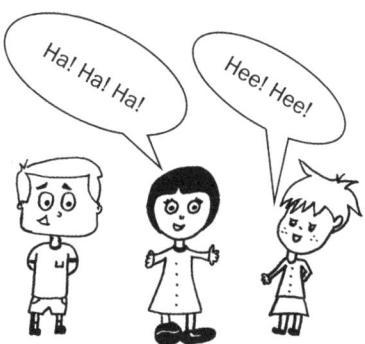

But no-one has ever laughed at Sophie when she speaks and her stutter is barely noticeable most of the time.

Sophie knows she doesn't have to speak at the school sports day, but she is still worried. 'What if I fall over and people laugh at me?' thinks Sophie as the school sports day is about to start. 'What if I drop my egg off the spoon and it rolls into the spectators and I can't get it back? What if no-one wants to be my partner in the three-legged race? What if I come last in the running race? Everyone will say mean things to me and think I'm useless. I'll never be able to go back to school and face them all again.'

Sophie is called to the start line for the egg and spoon race. All around her children have big happy smiles on their faces.

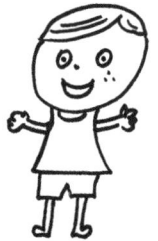 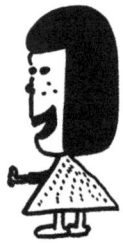 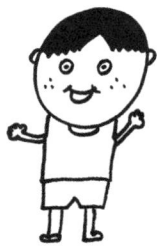

But Sophie is sweating and shaking so much she can barely hold the spoon. She feels so dizzy she has no idea how she is going to run. 'I'm so useless,' thinks Sophie. 'I can't do this!'

Sophie sees her parents and grandparents waving at her near the starting line. 'They are going to be so disappointed in me when I come last,' she thinks.

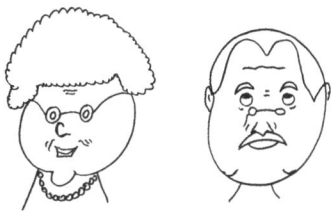

As the whistle blows for the race to start, all the other children begin running, spoons in hand. But Sophie just stands still and cries.

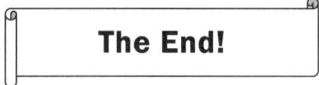

The End!

SOPHIE PICTURE A

Below is a picture of an anxious Sophie. Write some of the anxious thoughts that Sophie had about the school sports day in the thought bubble.

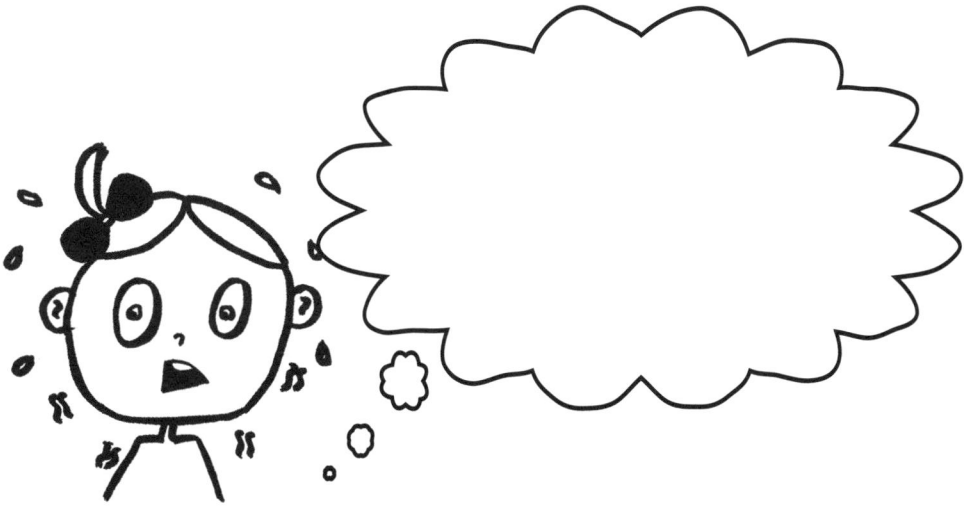

SOPHIE PICTURE B

Now we have a picture of a calm-looking Sophie because she has become a Thought Detective and has searched for the facts. Write some fact-based thoughts that Sophie could have about the school sports day in the speech bubble.

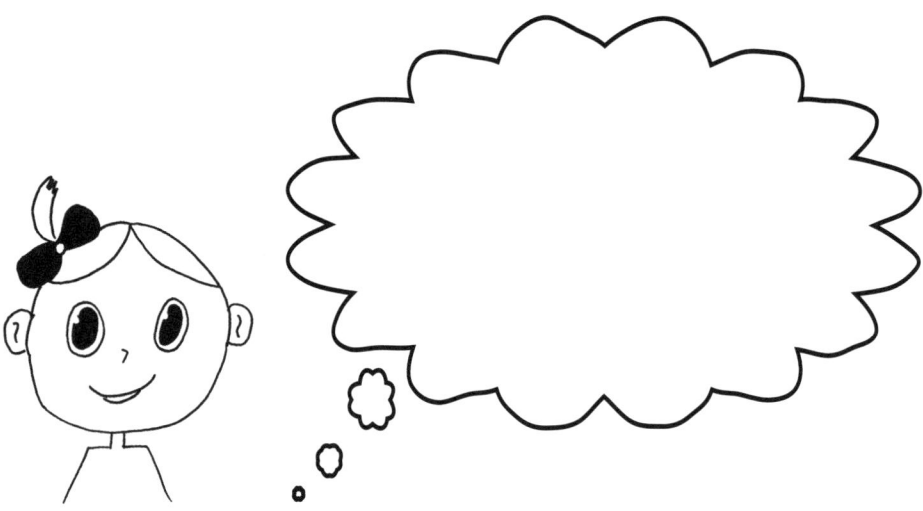

You might have written the following fact-based thoughts or ones that are similar:

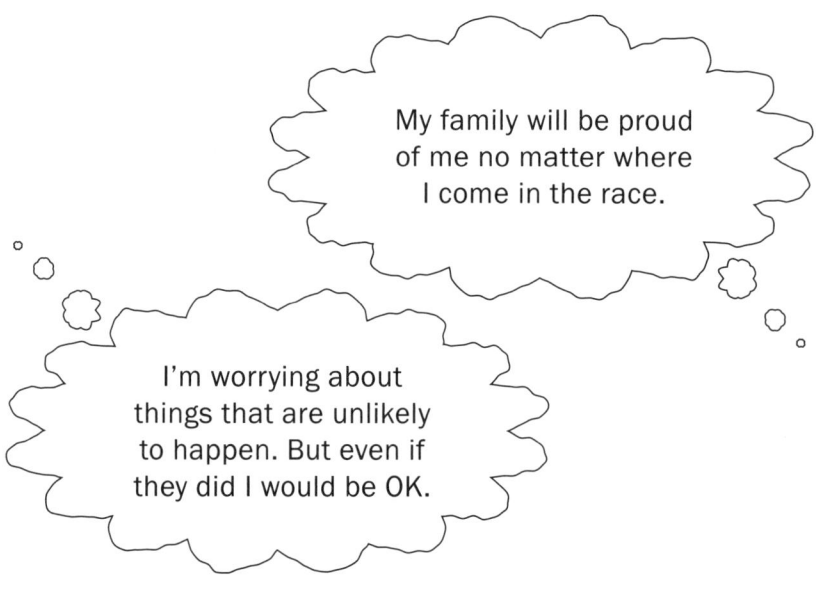

QUESTION: Which set of thoughts starve Sophie's Anxiety Gremlin? Circle your answer.

Thoughts in Sophie Picture A   Thoughts in Sophie Picture B

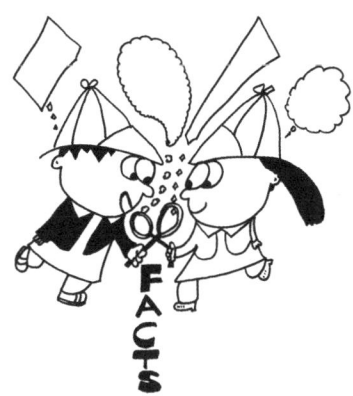

The thoughts in Sophie Picture B starve her Anxiety Gremlin because she is searching for the facts like a good Thought Detective. But the thoughts in Sophie Picture A are coming through her Anxiety Thinking Glasses. By thinking that way she is feeding her Anxiety Gremlin.

So whenever you find yourself feeling anxious you can starve your Anxiety Gremlin by:

- ditching your Anxiety Thinking Glasses!
- being a Thought Detective searching for the facts!

IMPORTANT FACTS THAT ALL THOUGHT DETECTIVES NEED TO KNOW!

The first set of important facts that ALL Thought Detectives need to know are...

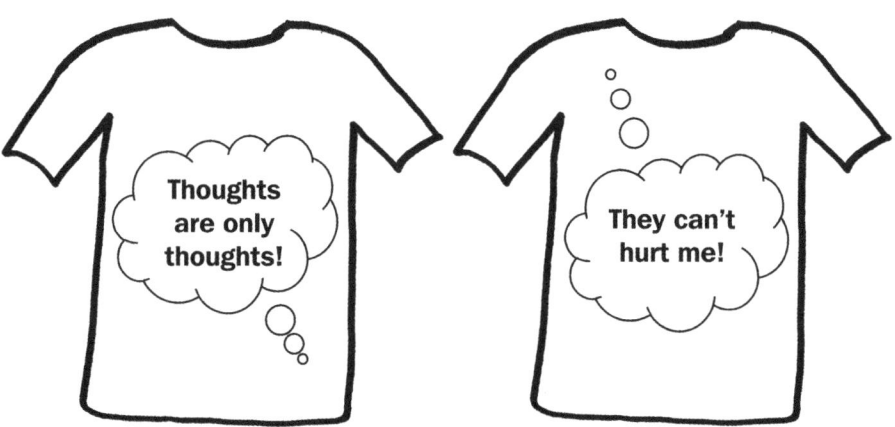

So it doesn't matter how many anxious thoughts you have whizzing through your head, they cannot hurt you. They are only thoughts!

The second set of facts that ALL Thought Detectives need to search for are...

facts about themselves.

Searching for these facts will help you to ditch the following Anxiety Thinking Glasses:

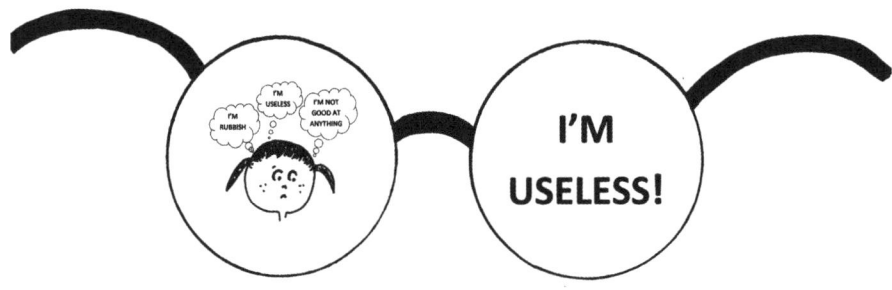

I'm Useless! Glasses

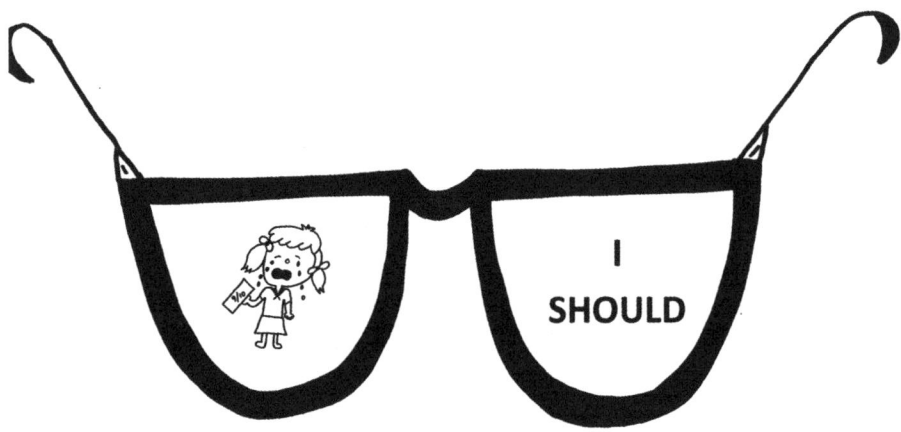

I Should Glasses

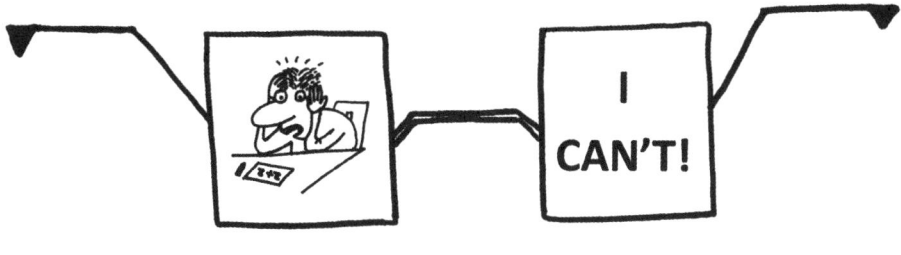

I Can't! Glasses

By finding out the facts about yourself, you will realise that:

- you have many good qualities, skills and talents that you should be very proud of!
- you don't have to be perfect as everyone makes mistakes and that is OK!
- you can do more than you give yourself credit for!

One way to search for these facts as a Thought Detective is to create an...

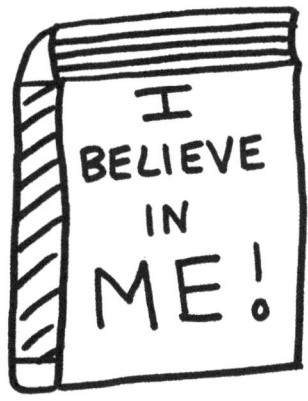

I Believe in Me! Book

An **I Believe in Me! Book** is the place that you can write all the facts that you learn about yourself that show you good things about you, such as:

- your good qualities
- things you are good at
- your skills and talents
- things that make you a good friend
- things that make you a good son/daughter or brother/sister
- things that you have achieved.

Try making your own **I Believe in Me! Book**. Design it however you like and fill it with all the great facts about you!

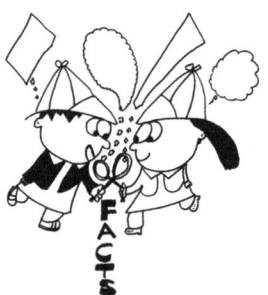

Now you have learnt about different ways to become a great Thought Detective and to ditch your Anxiety Thinking Glasses, draw a picture of yourself as a Thought Detective searching for the facts and ditching your Anxiety Thinking Glasses in the box below!

Me as a Thought Detective!

Act Differently

As you saw in Chapter 8, when we get anxious we can often act in ways that aren't good for us. But we don't have to avoid situations or hide from people as those things feed your Anxiety Gremlin! You have a choice to act differently. Here is a story to explain what I mean.

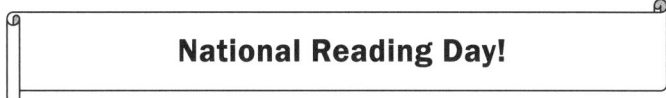

National Reading Day!

The school bell rings and all the children in Hope Street School file into the school assembly one by one and sit on the floor.

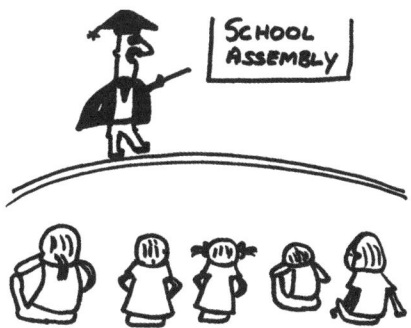

'Today's assembly is to celebrate National Reading Day,' says Headmaster Jones. Seven-year-old Grant loves to read and is an excellent reader. So his teacher Mrs Wilson has picked him to stand up in the school assembly and read in front of everyone.

Grant may love to read, but he hates reading in front of other people. He is afraid of making mistakes as Grant believes he should be perfect at everything he does.

When it's his turn to read, Grant walks to the front of the stage. His heart beats really fast in his chest and he feels like he can't breathe properly. He turns to face the audience, book in hand.

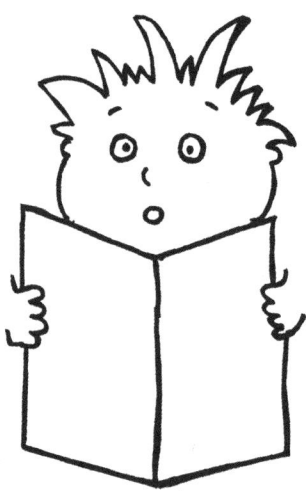

But as he looks at all the faces in front of him, Grant drops the book on the stage and runs from the hall!

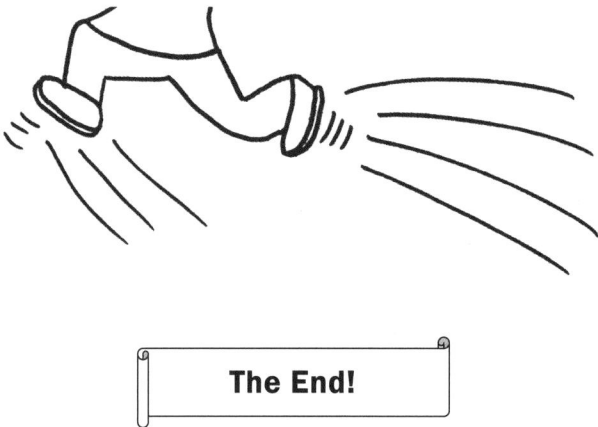

The End!

QUESTION: Did Grant's behaviour starve or feed his Anxiety Gremlin? Circle your answer.

Starve his Anxiety Gremlin   Feed his Anxiety Gremlin

Now draw a picture of how you think Grant could have acted differently in the box below. It needs to be a behaviour which would have had better results for him and made him feel less anxious.

How Grant could have acted differently

QUESTION: Would this behaviour starve or feed Grant's Anxiety Gremlin?

Starve his Anxiety Gremlin   Feed his Anxiety Gremlin

How to Act Differently to Starve Your Anxiety Gremlin

Here are some ways to act differently when you feel anxious to help you starve your Anxiety Gremlin! Grant could have done some of these!

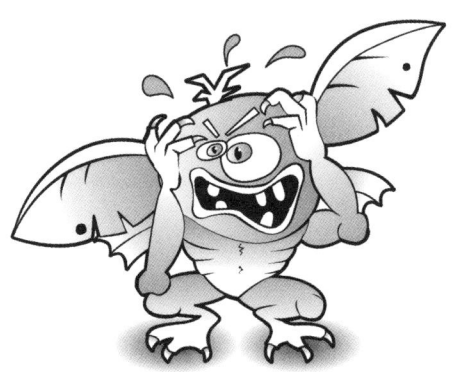

Talk

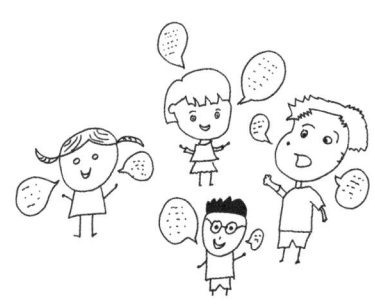

You can talk to someone that you trust, like a teacher, about how you are feeling. They can help you to become a Thought Detective and search for the facts. They can also help you to work out what to do to resolve any problem that may have led you to be anxious.

Create a Worry Box

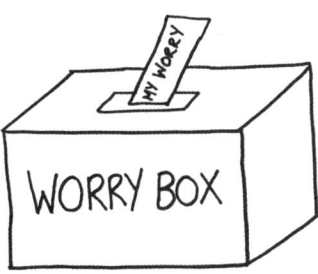

You can draw or write down the things that you get anxious about and put them in a Worry Box. Then when you feel calmer you can take them out and be a Thought Detective and search for the facts. If you realise there is no longer any need to be anxious about those things, you can throw the pieces of paper away along with your anxiety!

Why not have a go at making your own Worry Box? You can design and decorate it how you like!

Fill in a Worry Diary

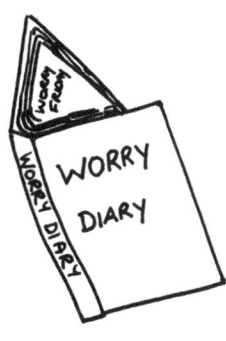

Often writing or drawing about your anxiety can help you to be a Thought Detective and search for the facts. It can also help you to work out what you can do to resolve a problem or how you can act better next time a similar thing happens. You will find an example diary on the next page.

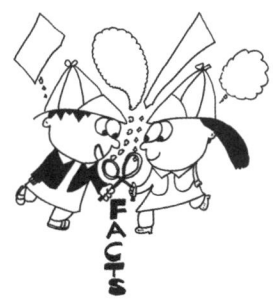

Anxiety Diary

Write or draw your answers to the following questions in the spaces below.

Date . . . .

What did you get anxious about today?

What were your thoughts?

Did you think through Anxiety Thinking Glasses? Circle your answer.

        Yes   No

What anxious physical feelings did you have?

Copyright © Kate Collins-Donnelly 2014

How did you act?

What effects did your anxiety have on you?

Which of the following did you do? Circle your answer.

Starve your Anxiety Gremlin   Feed your Anxiety Gremlin

If you fed him, what could you have done differently to starve him?

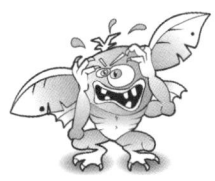

Problem solve

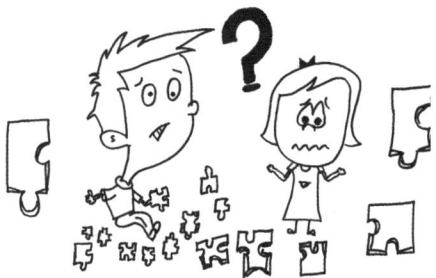

It is better to try and deal with a problem instead of getting more and more anxious about it! Ask yourself three questions to help you do this:

1. What is the problem that I am anxious about?

2. What things could I do about it?

3. Which would bring the best results and starve my Anxiety Gremlin?

Worry time

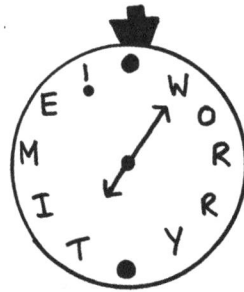

Worry time is a specific time in the day that you can use to talk, think, draw or write about your worries in the ways shown above. It is the time you can use to be a Thought Detective and work out how to resolve any problems you may have. But set a time limit for worry time as the less time you spend on your worries, the less you feed your Anxiety Gremlin.

Exercise

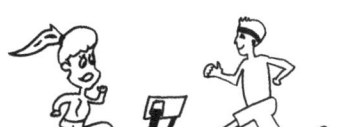

Exercise will help you to get rid of all those anxious physical feelings!

Relax

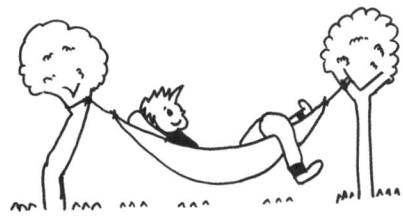

Take deep breaths and do things that make you feel chilled, such as reading a book, watching TV, listening to music or playing a game!

Visualise

This means picturing something that makes you feel calm or happy or something that makes you laugh in your head. This will help you feel calmer!

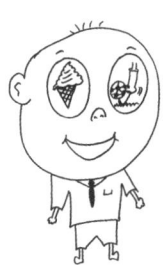

Distract yourself

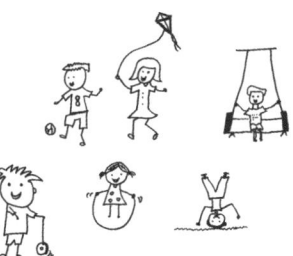

Distract yourself from feeling anxious by doing things that you enjoy!

Sleep

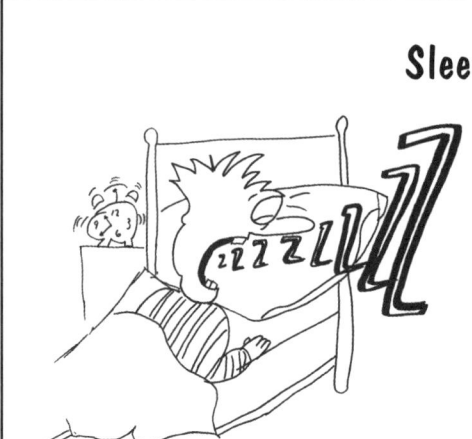

Getting enough sleep is really important! If we are too tired because we haven't slept enough, we can be more likely to get anxious.

Let's look at how some of these strategies might help you to starve your Anxiety Gremlin. You can write or draw your answers in the boxes below.

My choice of exercise would be...	My way to relax would be...

My way to distract myself would be…	**My happy or calm picture in my mind would be…**
My worry time would be at the following time…	**The person I would talk to about my feelings would be…**

Become a Behaviour Scientist!

A final way to starve your Anxiety Gremlin by acting differently is to become a Behaviour Scientist!

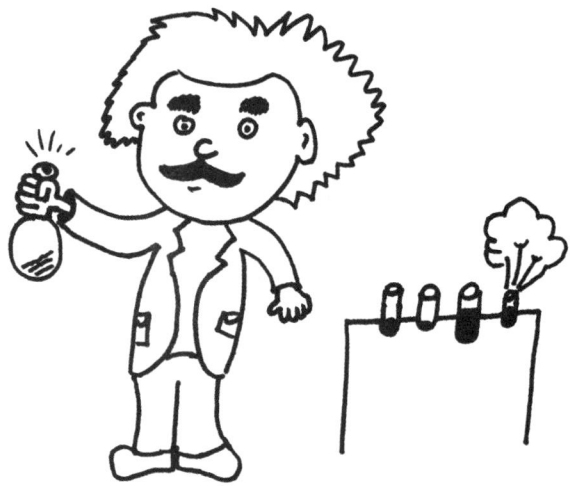

Do you remember how in Chapter 8 we said that when we get anxious we often act in ways that aren't good for us? Well, becoming a Behaviour Scientist will help you to stop acting in those ways bit by bit! You can design experiments that involve you slowly stopping the anxious behaviours that aren't good for you. Here's how!

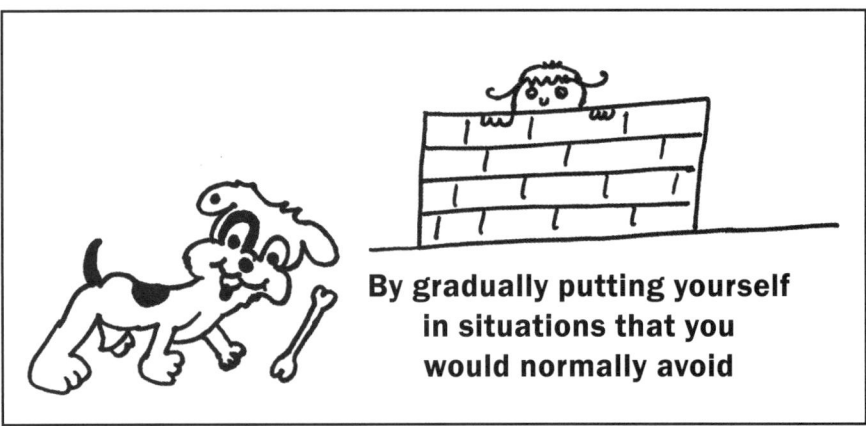

By gradually putting yourself in situations that you would normally avoid

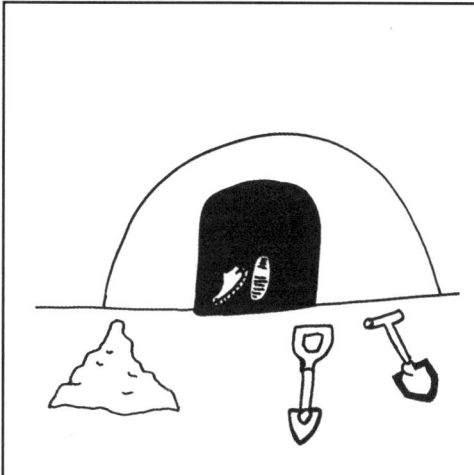

By gradually staying for longer periods of time in situations that you would normally escape from

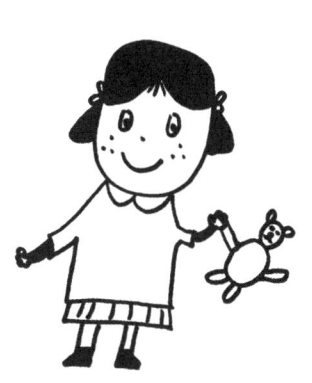

By gradually reducing the amount of time you have to have certain things with you for comfort

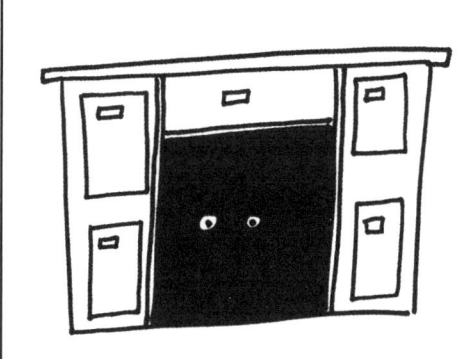

By gradually putting yourself in situations that you would normally hide from

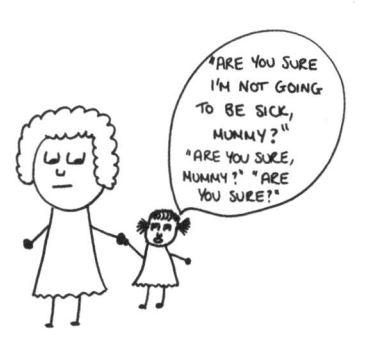

By gradually reducing the number of times you say certain words or ask people certain things

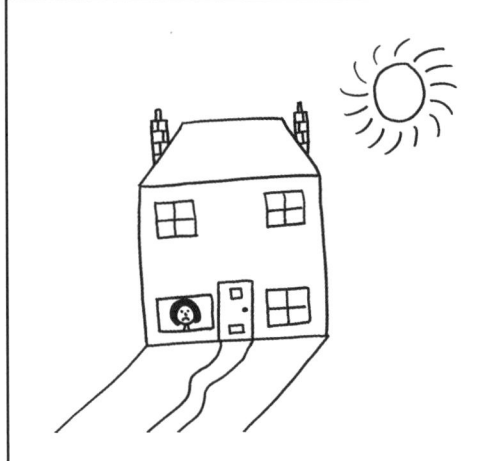

By leaving the house for longer and longer periods of time

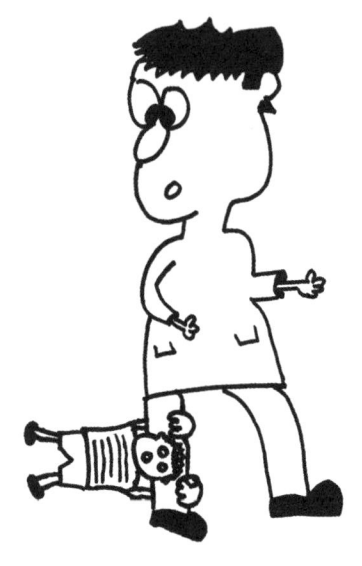

By gradually reducing the amount of time you have your parents by your side when it is safe to do so

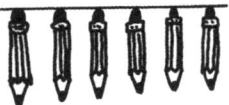

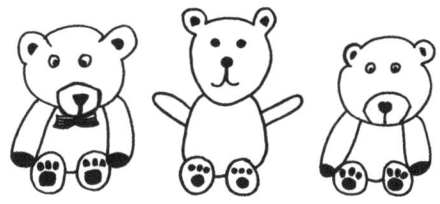

By gradually reducing the amount you wash, check, organise, tidy, count, touch or collect things

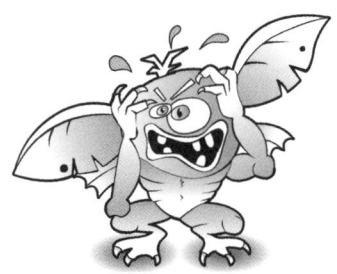

Starving the Anxiety Gremlin Strategies   155

When you stop acting in ways that aren't good for you, you get the chance to see that the situation wasn't as bad as you thought and you starve your Anxiety Gremlin!

Design an Experiment for Simon

Simon is nine years old and he is afraid of meat. He thinks if he goes into a room containing meat, he will become ill.

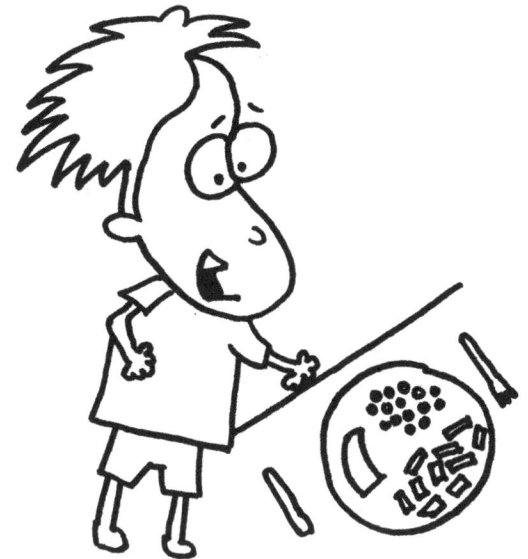

As a result, Simon avoids eating in the same room as his parents as they are meat eaters. He also avoids being in the kitchen when his parents cook meat and he avoids going in the school canteen as they serve meat.

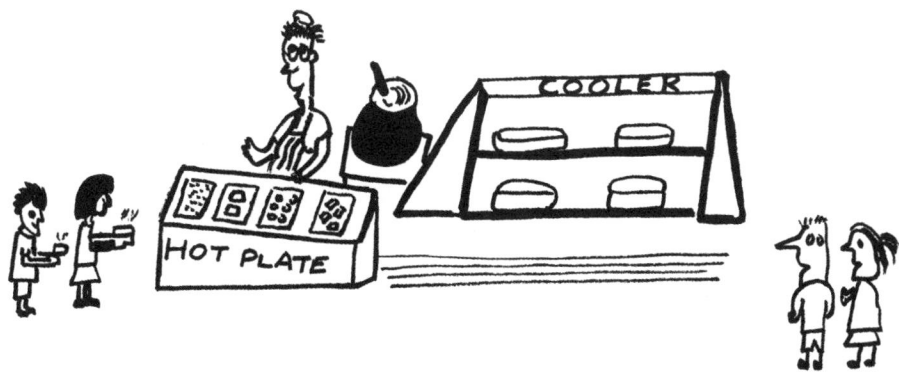

Write or draw a behaviour experiment for Simon in the box below.

A Behaviour Experiment for Simon

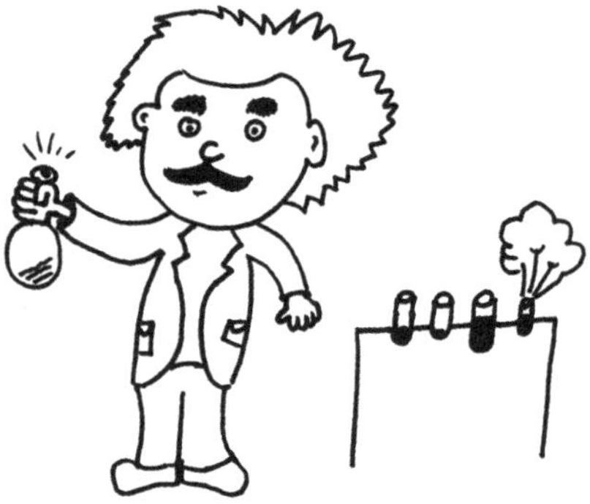

In the box on the next page design your own Behaviour Scientist Experiment to help you stop acting in ways that aren't good for you bit by bit. Then try carrying out the experiment step by step using all the other anxiety management strategies you have learnt in this chapter to help you keep calm along the way. You may feel very anxious when you first start the experiment, but as you complete each step, your Anxiety Gremlin will shrink and you will become less anxious over time! Good luck!

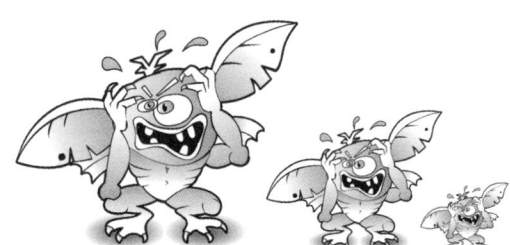

My Behaviour Experiment

Well done! You've completed Step 9 in starving your Anxiety Gremlin! You've done amazingly well! Be proud and colour in your ninth **Starving the Anxiety Gremlin Star**!

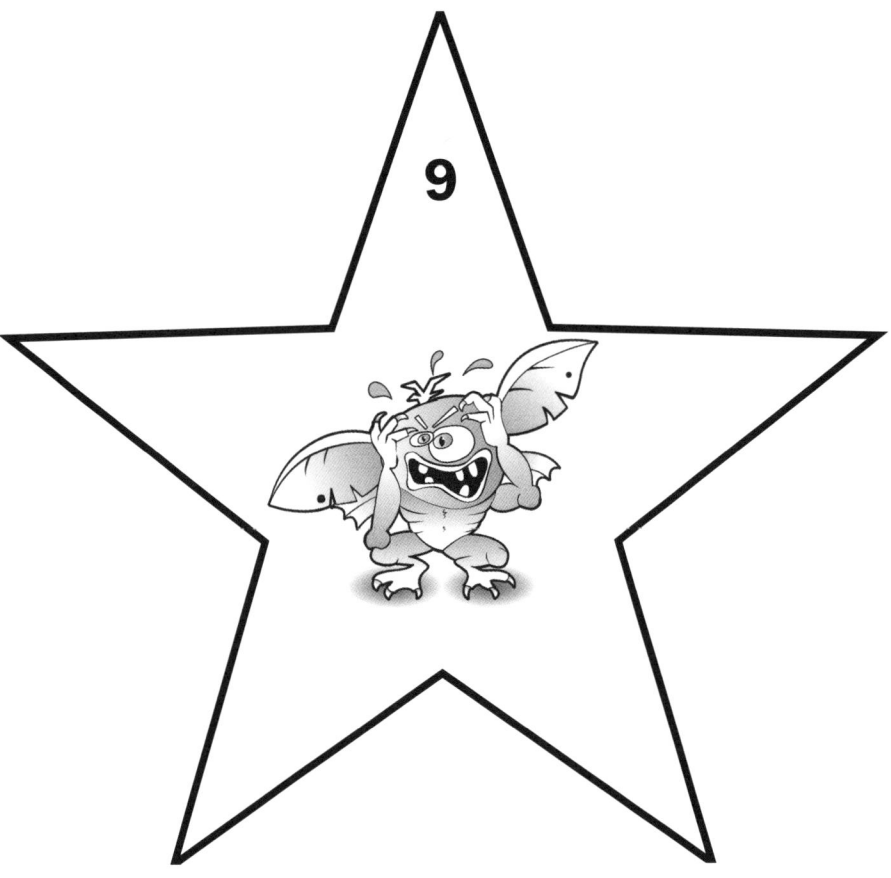

Now complete one or both of the following **Just for Fun Puzzles** as a reward! Enjoy!

Missing Piece!

A jigsaw piece is missing from the picture below. See if you can work out which piece it is. Circle your answer.

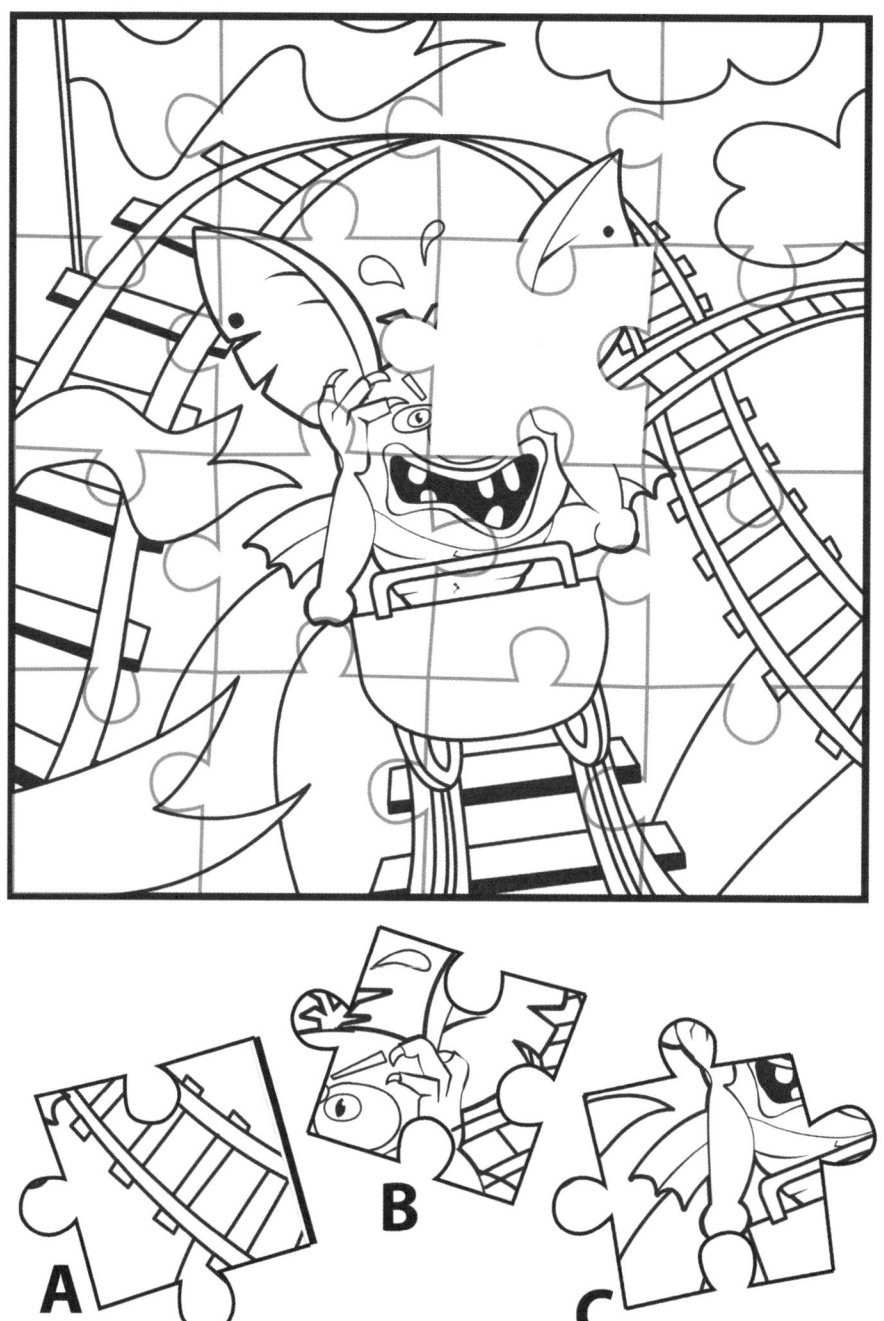

Starve the Anxiety Gremlin Fill-In Puzzle

Below are some of the ways to starve your Anxiety Gremlin. See if you can complete the puzzle below by fitting all the words into the crossword grid. Each word shares at least one letter with another word in the list.

HINT: Start with the 10-letter word!

3-Letter	4-Letter	5-Letter
BOX	TALK	SLEEP
	TIME	WRITE
		RELAX
		SOLVE
		DIARY
8-Letter	**9-Letter**	**10-Letter**
EXERCISE	VISUALISE	EXPERIMENT
DISTRACT	DETECTIVE	

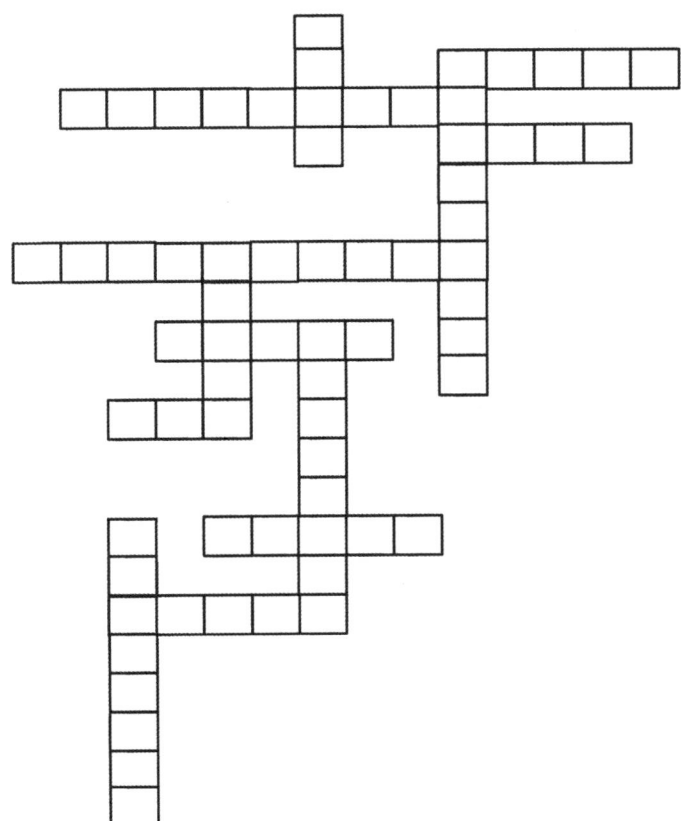

11

Your Anxiety Dos and Don'ts!

For the next two activities you'll need some paper, pens, crayons or paints and even some glue and glitter if you like!

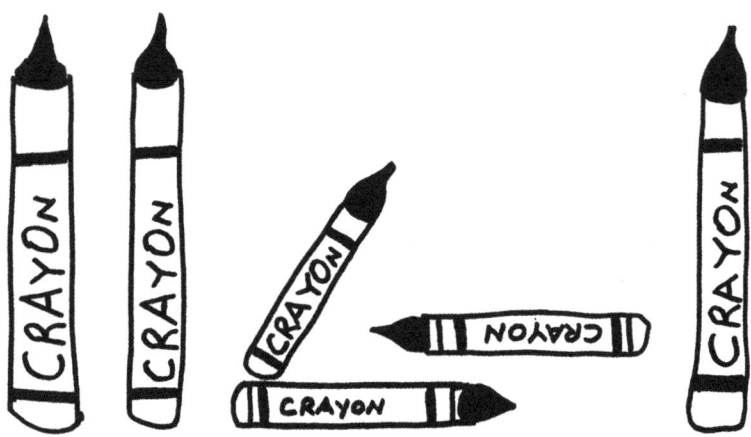

Anxiety Dos and Don'ts Chart

Now it's time for you to think about everything you have learnt throughout this book and create your own Anxiety Dos and Don'ts Chart. Try and come up with at least five of each. Remember the Dos will be things that starve your Anxiety Gremlin!

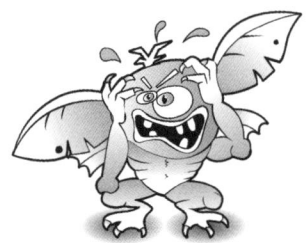

It can help to have one of these pinned up somewhere at home so you can look at it and remind yourself of what you need to do to starve your Anxiety Gremlin. You can even make a second one to keep in your school bag!

Have fun creating your chart and decorate it however you like. Use your imagination!

Well done! I bet your Dos and Don'ts Chart looks great! Completing this chart was Step 10 in your mission to starve your Anxiety Gremlin. Colour in your tenth **Starving the Anxiety Gremlin Star** to celebrate!

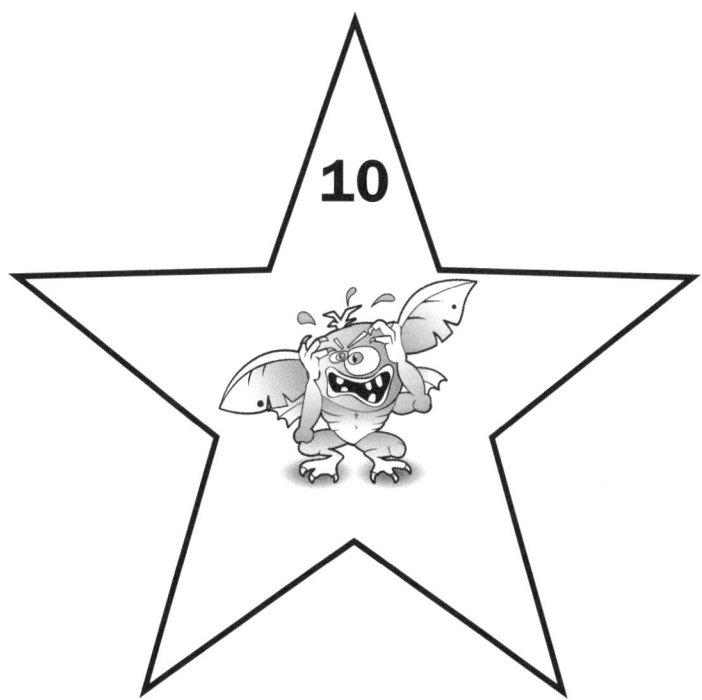

Now complete one or both of the following **Just for Fun Puzzles** as a reward for having learnt so much about how to starve your Anxiety Gremlin! Enjoy!

Memory Game!

- STEP A: Read through your Dos and Don'ts Chart for one minute.
- STEP B: Cover up your chart and see how many dos and don'ts you can remember in one minute!

Good luck!

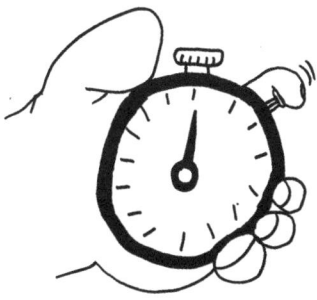

Crack the Code!

Below is an important message written in code. You need to crack this code to reveal its hidden message! I've told you what some of the symbols mean but not all of them. Happy code breaking!

THE MESSAGE

1 * △ 2 □ 3

@ 4 2

△ 5 7 ⌂ 3 * #

+ 2 3 ? 6 ⌂ 5

THE CODE

1 = S	2 = R	3 = ___
4 = ___	5 = ___	6 = ___
7 = ___	△ = A	? = M
⌂ = I	# = Y	+ = G
* = ___	□ = ___	@ = ___

12
Completing Your Mission to Starve the Anxiety Gremlin!

Congratulations! You have now learnt all you need to know about anxiety and how to starve your Anxiety Gremlin. It's now down to you to put it into practice. This is the final step in your mission to starve your Anxiety Gremlin. Remember...

You are in control of your anxiety!

You can choose to starve your Anxiety Gremlin!

Here is a quiz to help you recap on everything you have learnt throughout this workbook.

The Anxiety Quiz

1. **Fill in the blank. Another word for a feeling is an E _ _ _ _ _**

2. **Colour in the odd one out. HINT: The odd one out is not a feeling!**

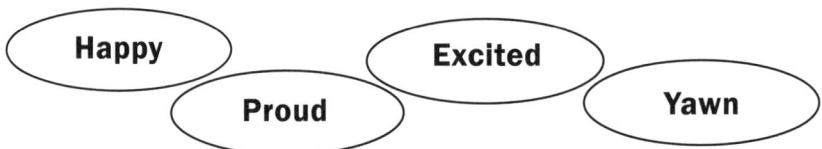

3. **Name two feelings beginning with the letter 'S'. HINT: Take a look at these two faces!**

4. **Unscramble the word. Anxiety is a GLEFENI.**

    F _ _ _ _ _ _

5. **It is normal to worry occasionally. Circle the correct answer.**

    True   False

6. **Anxiety is when you experience which three feelings too often? Tick the correct answer.**

    a. Worry, fear and nervousness ☐
    b. Anger, surprise and jealousy ☐
    c. Happiness, joy and excitement ☐

7. **Fill in the blank. Fight or F_ _ _ _ _ response**

8. **Unscramble these anxiety triggers.**

    a. LACPES   P _ _ _ _ _
    b. PEEPLO   P _ _ _ _ _
    c. NMILAAS   A _ _ _ _ _ _
    d. SITNUAIOTS   S _ _ _ _ _ _ _ _

9. **Fill in the blank. Anxiety Thinking G _ _ _ _ _ _**

10. **Which of these are anxious behaviours that are bad for you? Tick your answers.**

    a. Avoid ☐
    b. Escape ☐
    c. Relax ☐
    d. Problem solve ☐

11. **Which of these are physical feelings of anxiety? Tick your answers.**

    a. Sweating ☐
    b. Shaking ☐
    c. Feeling dizzy ☐
    d. Blowing your nose ☐

12. **Who is in control of your anxiety? Tick the correct answer.**

    a. You ☐
    b. Your parents ☐
    c. Your dog ☐
    d. The Anxiety Gremlin ☐

13. **What do you need to do to the Anxiety Gremlin? Tick the correct answer.**

    a. Starve it ☐
    b. Feed it ☐
    c. Hug it ☐

14. **Which of these are ways to starve the Anxiety Gremlin? Tick your answers.**

    a. Talk ☐
    b. Distract yourself ☐
    c. Be a Thought Detective ☐
    d. Hide ☐
    e. Think through Anxiety Thinking Glasses ☐

I'm sure you will have done great on the quiz! Well done!

Has Your Anxiety Changed?

Here are some questions to help you see if your anxiety has changed in any way as you have worked through this book. I've asked you most of these questions before earlier in this workbook. I have introduced three new questions as well.

QUESTION 1

How often do you get anxious? Circle your answer.

Most of the time   Often   Sometimes

Rarely   Never

QUESTION 2

Below are some negative anxious behaviours pictures. Circle any that you still do when you get anxious.

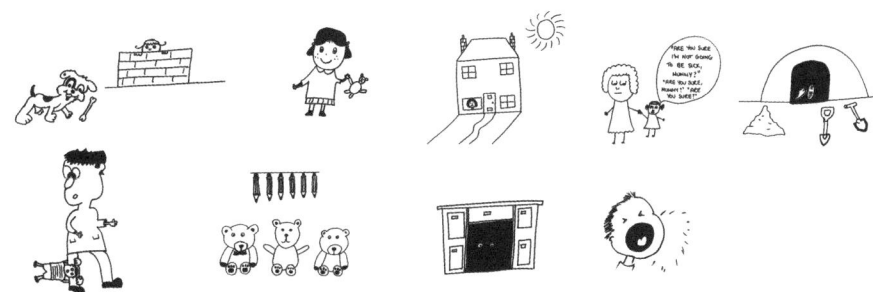

QUESTION 3

Here are some pictures of the different bad effects that anxiety can have. Circle or colour in the pictures that show how your anxiety is still affecting you.

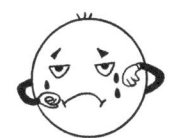
Feeling sad, unhappy, guilty, angry or ashamed

Feeling poorly
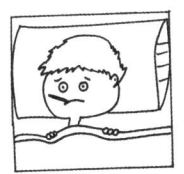

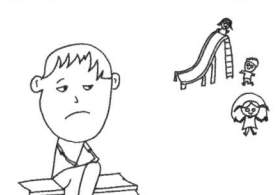
Feeling lonely

| Feeling useless 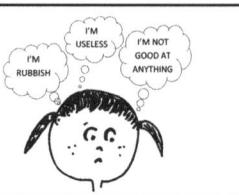 |

|  Getting lower grades at school |

| Missing out on fun or important things 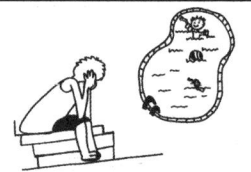 |

QUESTION 4

Do you now do any of the following to starve your Anxiety Gremlin?

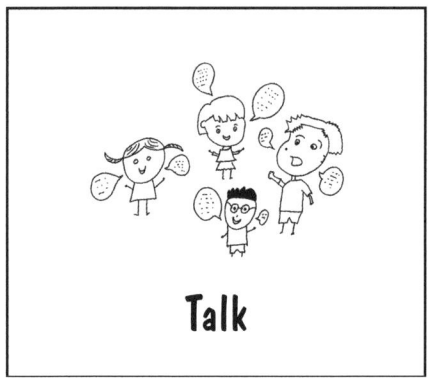

Talk

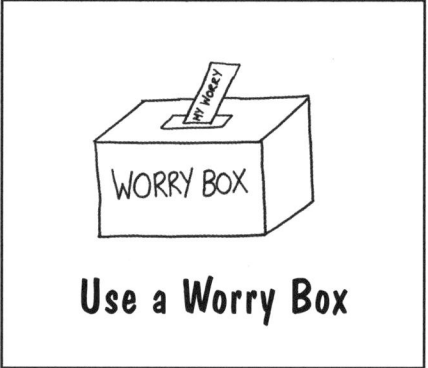

Use a Worry Box

Completing Your Mission to Starve the Anxiety Gremlin 171

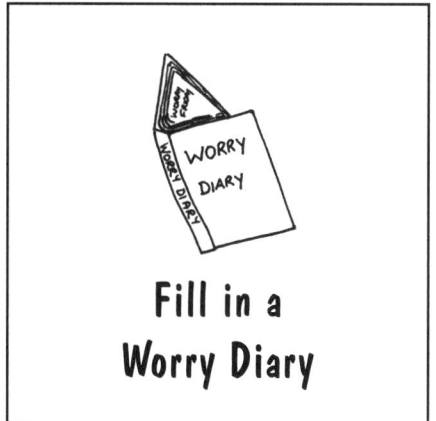

Fill in a Worry Diary

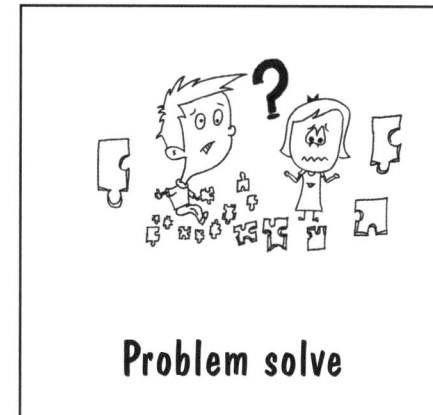

Problem solve

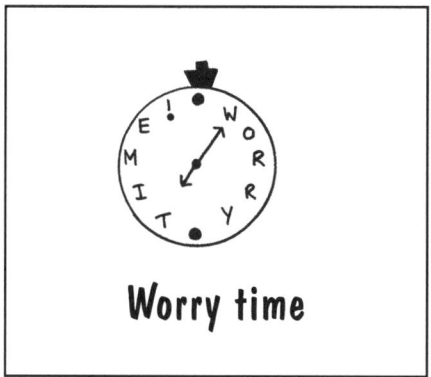

Worry time

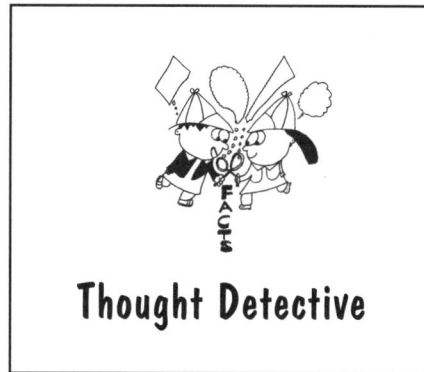

Thought Detective

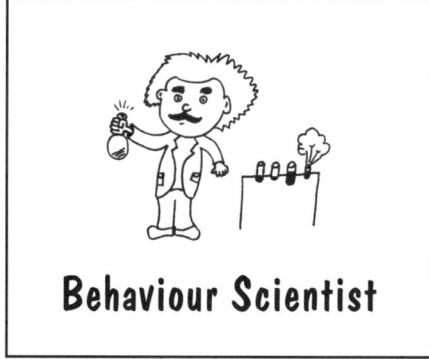

Behaviour Scientist

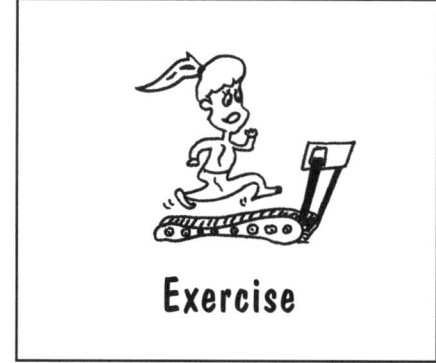

Exercise

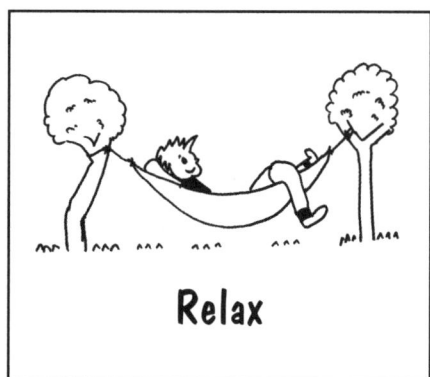

Relax

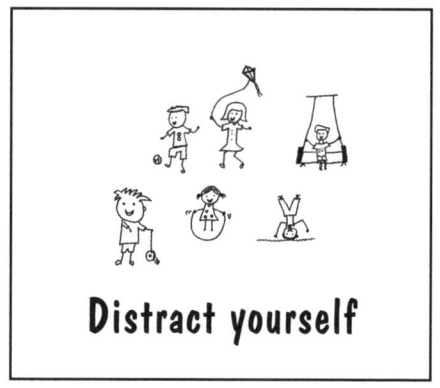

Distract yourself

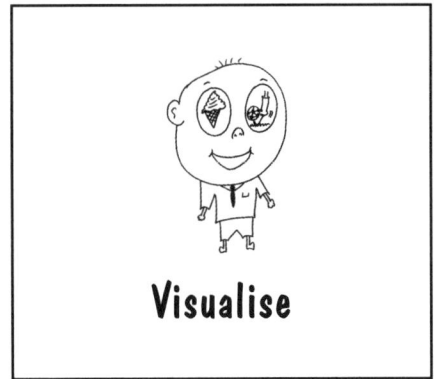

Visualise

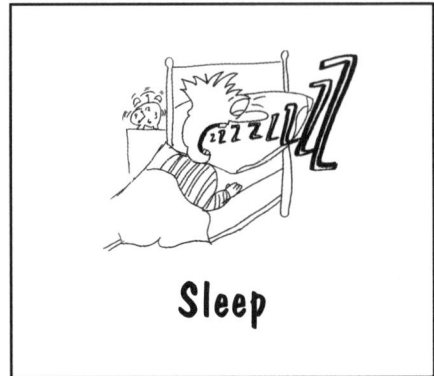

Sleep

QUESTION 5

Colour in your answer. Since starting this book...

| I haven't starved my Anxiety Gremlin at all | I have starved my Anxiety Gremlin a little | I have starved my Anxiety Gremlin a lot |

QUESTION 6

Colour in your answer. Since starting this book my anxiety has...

| Got less | Stayed the same | Got worse |

What You Have Learnt

Now let's look at what you feel you have learnt by completing this workbook. Tick the box for each item that you feel you have learnt.

I understand what feelings are. ☐

I understand that it is normal to feel worried, nervous or scared occasionally. ☐

I understand that anxiety occurs when we get worried, nervous or afraid too often. ☐

I understand what the fight or flight response is. ☐

I can name different types of anxiety triggers. ☐

I am aware of some of my own anxiety triggers. ☐

I can name some anxious physical feelings. ☐

I am aware of some of my own anxious physical feelings. ☐

I can name some ways that people might act when they get anxious that aren't good for them. ☐

I am aware of some of my own anxious behaviours that aren't good for me. ☐

I understand that it's how I think about a situation that leads me to be anxious, not the situation itself. ☐

I understand what feeds my Anxiety Gremlin.

I understand the types of thoughts that feed my Anxiety Gremlin. ☐

I understand what Anxiety Thinking Glasses are. ☐

I understand the types of behaviours that feed my Anxiety Gremlin. ☐

I understand that if I feed my Anxiety Gremlin too often my anxiety will get worse. ☐

I understand that feeding my Anxiety Gremlin too often can have bad effects on me and I can name some of these effects. ☐

I understand that I am in control of my anxiety. ☐

I understand that I can choose to starve my Anxiety Gremlin. ☐

I am aware of different ways to starve my Anxiety Gremlin. ☐

I understand what being a Thought Detective means. ☐

I understand what being a Behaviour Scientist means. ☐

I hope you have found that you have learnt lots and that your anxiety has started to improve. Here is your final **Starving the Anxiety Gremlin Star** as a reward for everything you have learnt and achieved. Congratulations! You should be so proud of yourself as you have worked incredibly hard! Have fun colouring in your star and remember you can keep collecting these stars as you work on starving your Anxiety Gremlin!

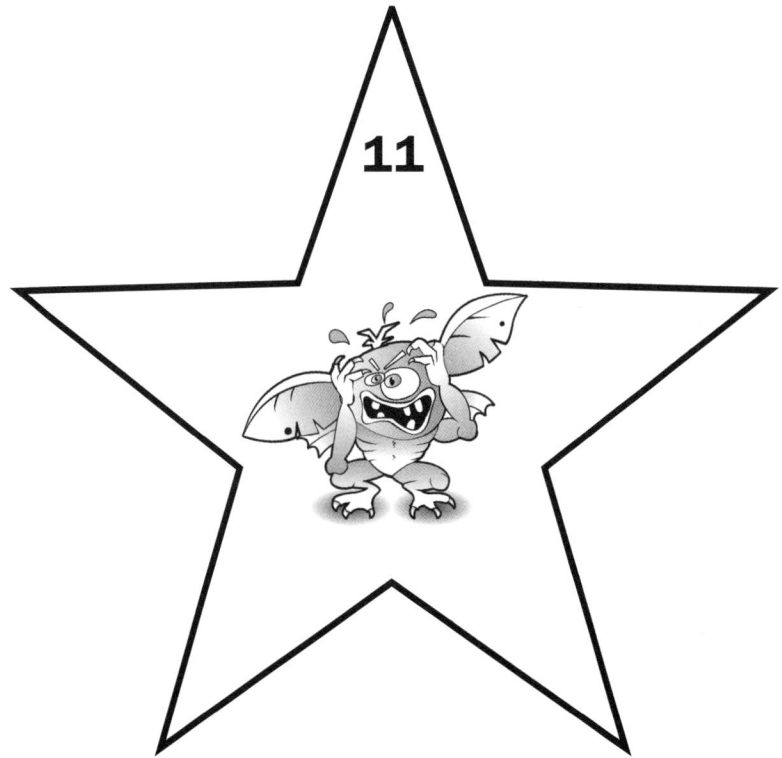

And here is your final **Just For Fun Puzzle** as a final reward! Enjoy!

The Anxiety Gremlin Fact-File!

This fact-file contains all the facts that you have learnt about the Anxiety Gremlin. But some of the words are missing. Try and fill in the blanks! And then colour in your final Anxiety Gremlin picture!

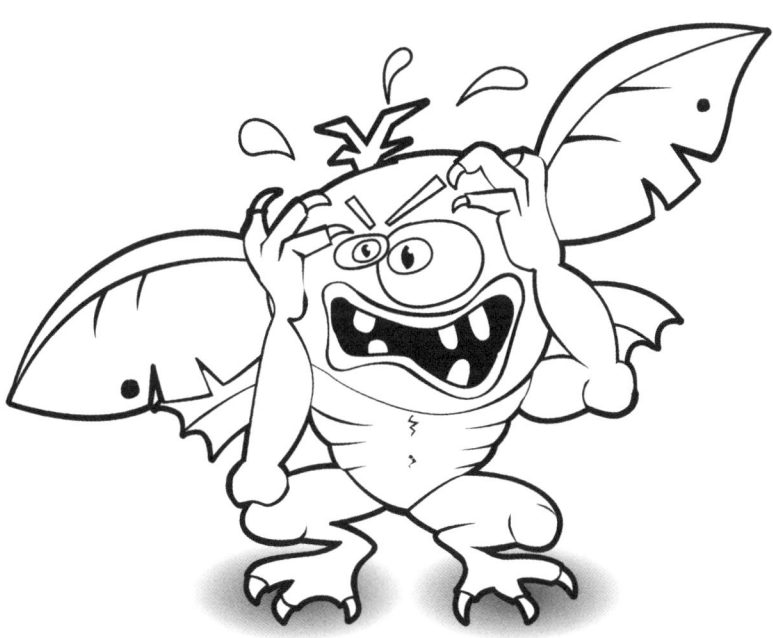

The Anxiety G __ __ __ __ __ __ is a troublesome pest.

The Anxiety Gremlin loves it when you get A __ __ __ __ __ __

If you think through Anxiety Thinking Glasses, you F __ __ __ the Anxiety Gremlin.

Anxious physical F __ __ __ __ __ __ __ feed the Anxiety Gremlin.

Anxious behaviours that are bad for you feed the A _ _ _ _ _ _ Gremlin.

The more you F _ _ _ the Anxiety Gremlin, the bigger he gets.

The B _ _ _ _ _ the Anxiety Gremlin gets, the more anxious you get.

The more anxious you get, the more bad effects your A _ _ _ _ _ _ has on you.

And the A _ _ _ _ _ _ Gremlin gets even bigger!

But if you think differently and A _ _ differently, you can starve the Anxiety Gremlin.

If you are a T _ _ _ _ _ _ Detective, you starve the Anxiety Gremlin.

If you are a Behaviour S _ _ _ _ _, you starve the Anxiety Gremlin.

If you S _ _ _ _ _ the Anxiety Gremlin, he will get smaller and smaller and you will get less and less anxious!

Good luck with starving your Anxiety Gremlin!

You can do it!

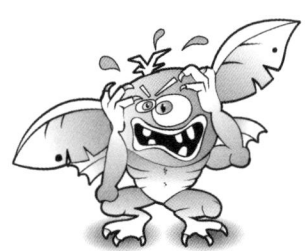

And here is a story from a young person who wants you to know that it is possible to starve the Anxiety Gremlin!

Dear Reader,

At my sixth birthday party I was sick. From then on I was very scared of being sick. Worrying about it made me shake and cry and upset my tummy. I didn't like eating and sometimes I couldn't sleep. I thought my worries would never go away. I did not want to go to school. I did not want to leave my house in case there was no toilet nearby. I didn't know anyone else who worried like I did. I felt all alone. I thought I was weird.

I didn't know what to do and Mum and Dad didn't know how to help me. So we went to see some people who can help with worries. They told me I could get rid of them.

At first it was hard. Things did not get better straight away and I had good days and bad days. But I learned to turn bad thoughts into good ones. I learned to breathe slowly when I got really scared. I kept a diary and wrote down how I felt. I told my Mum and Dad and friends when I was having a bad day. This helped. I learnt I wasn't weird and I wasn't the only person who worries.

I'm 17 now. I still worry sometimes because everyone does. But I don't worry a lot about being sick and I don't get really scared. And because I worry less, life is more fun. This book can help you to achieve this too.

So if you are feeling worried and scared, tell people how you are feeling so they can help you. I promise it gets better. Don't forget you are not alone, you aren't weird and most of all you are very very brave. And you can starve your Anxiety Gremlin just like I did!

Lots of love

Chloe :) xxx

This is to certify that

....

has successfully completed the
Starving the Anxiety Gremlin
workbook and can expertly

STARVE THEIR ANXIETY GREMLIN!

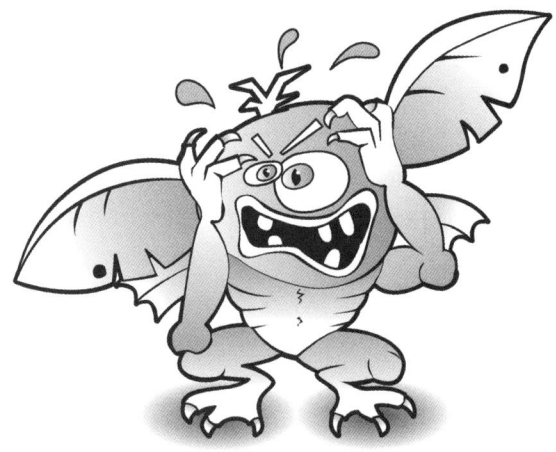

Activity, Puzzle and Quiz Answers

Escape the Anxiety Gremlin!

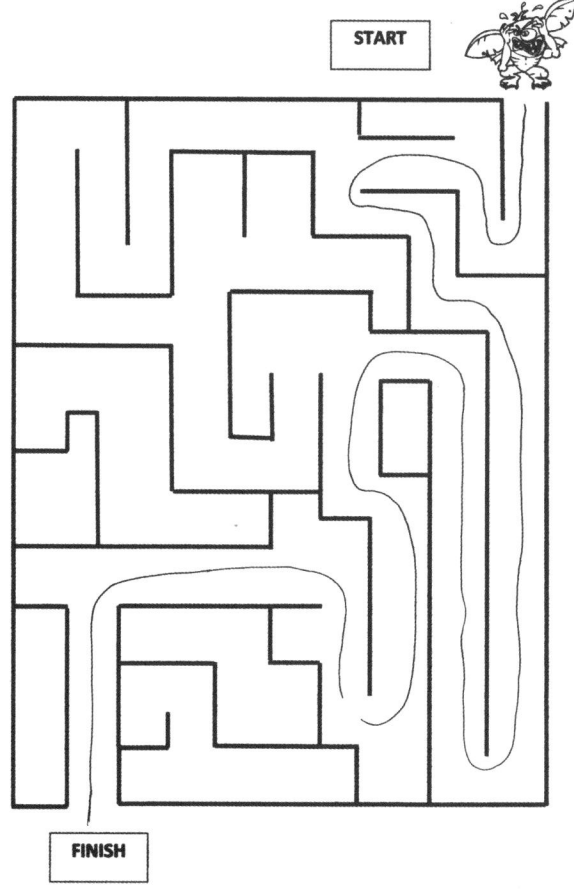

Gremlins Galore!

There are 30 Anxiety Gremlins in the hexagon.

Word Multiplication!

Some of the words you might have spotted include germ, green, the, anxiety, gremlin, linger, grim, men, rant, hat, heat, line…and the list goes on and on!

Feelings or Not Feelings? You Decide!

The feelings are guilty, upset, calm, relaxed, surprised, jealous, disappointed and unhappy.

Find the Feelings!

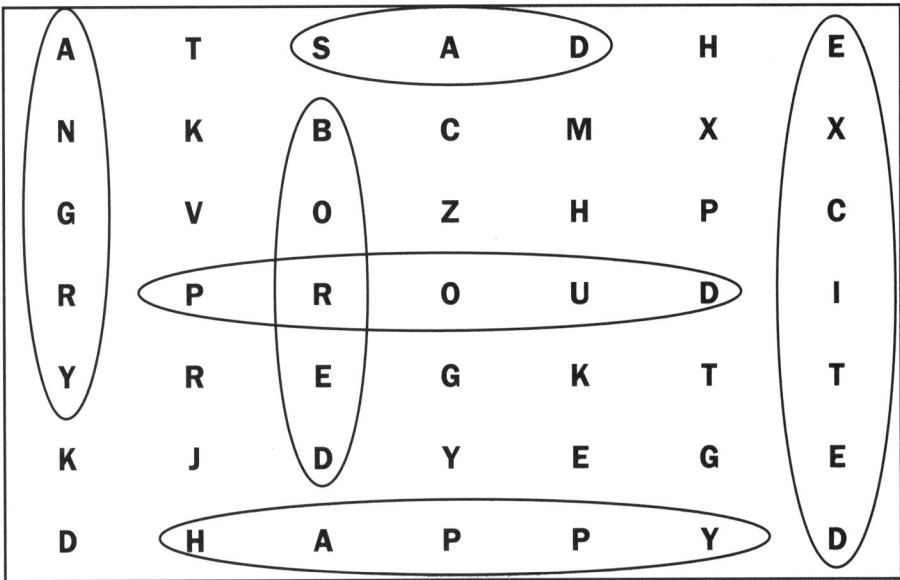

The Face and Feeling Mix-Up!

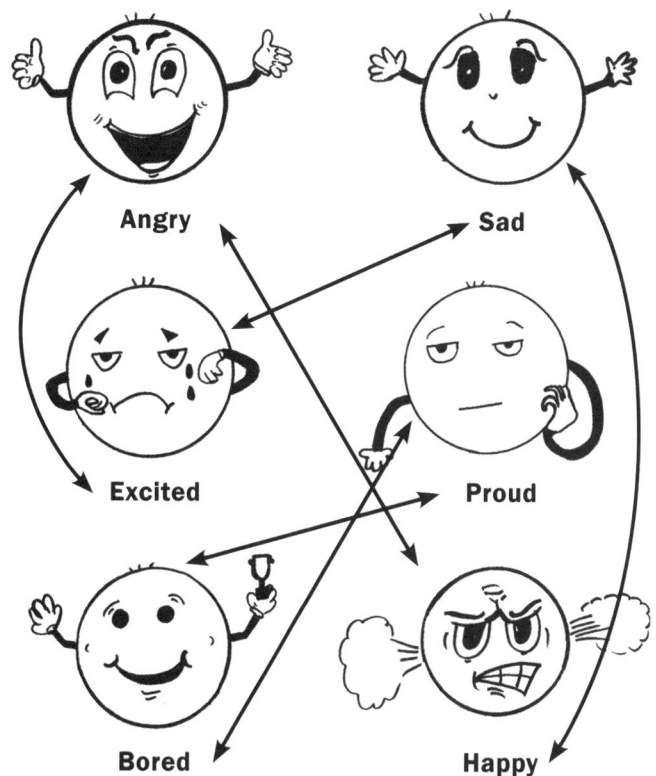

What Am I? Riddle

The answer is 'Feelings'.

The Anxious Feelings Spiral

The words are worry, nervousness and fear.

Go Dotty!

The picture reveals the Anxiety Gremlin!

Word Hunt

The word 'anxiety' appears five times.

Find the Pairs!

The names that go with the pictures in order of right to left on each line are: Tim, Ben, Fiona, Mandy, Nicholas, Neela, Abdul, Wesley, Max, Greg, Sally, Melissa, Carla, Grace, David, Helen, Lucy, Freddie.

How Many Gremlins?

There are ten Anxiety Gremlins in this chapter.

Odd Gremlin Out

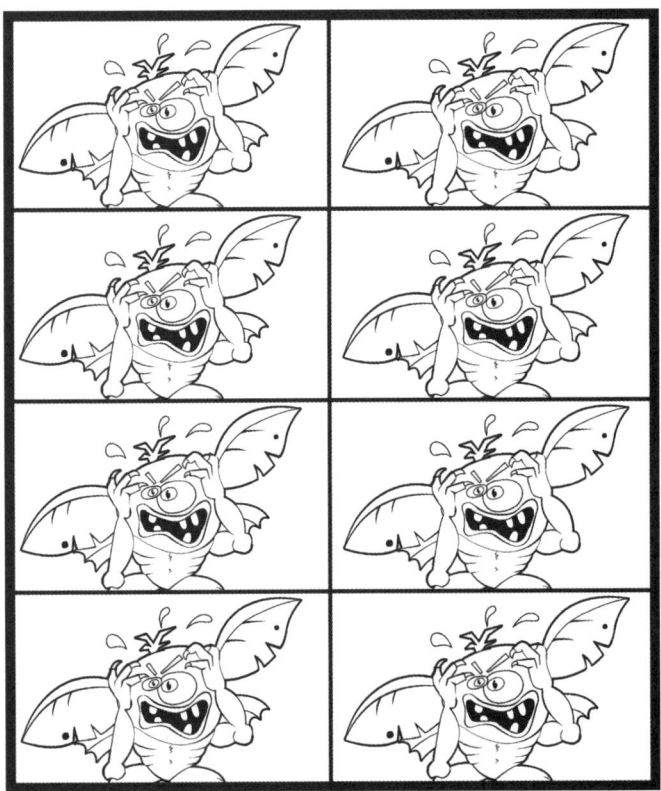

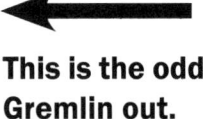

This is the odd Gremlin out.

Activity, Puzzle and Quiz Answers

Match Four!

The four matching Gremlins are marked with an X.

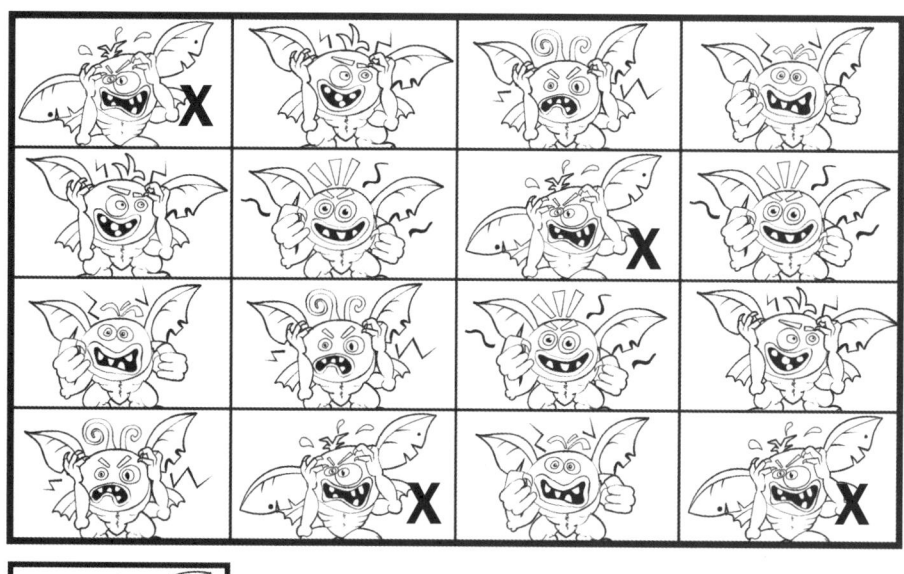

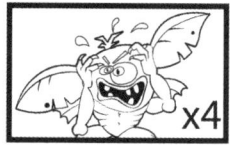

Word Jigsaw

THE	BIGG	ER Y	OUR
ANXI	ETY	GREM	LIN
THE	MORE	ANXI	OUS
	YOU	ARE	

I Spy Scramble!

The pictures are: fast breathing, stomach ache, knot in stomach, shaking, fast heart beat, headache, sweating, red face, butterflies in stomach, hot, cold, rash.

There are three physical feelings beginning with the letter 'S'.

A Physical Match

The labels on the pictures should read as follows from right to left on each line: hard to breathe, can't sleep, dizzy, feeling or being sick, jelly legs, lump in throat, go to the toilet a lot, not hungry, tired, tears, nightmares.

The Anxiety Gremlin Goes Line Dancing!

The answer is A.

Spot the Difference

The differences are marked with an X.

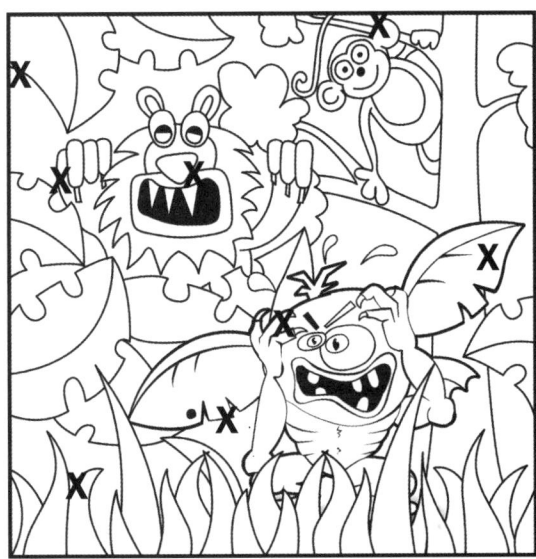

Find the Missing Letters

The sentence is:

Your Anxiety Gremlin will get bigger if you avoid things when you are anxious.

Hidden Gremlins

The Gremlins are marked with an X.

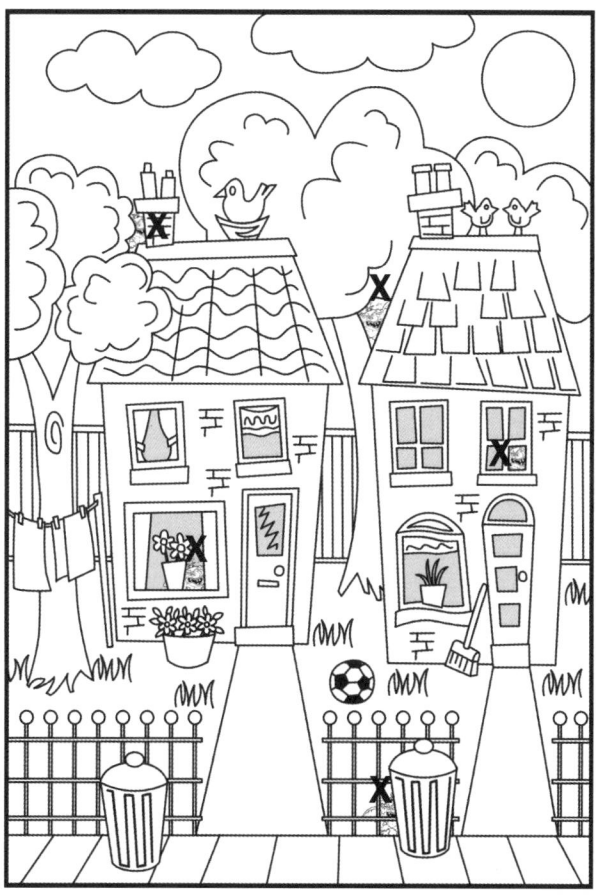

Picture Suduko

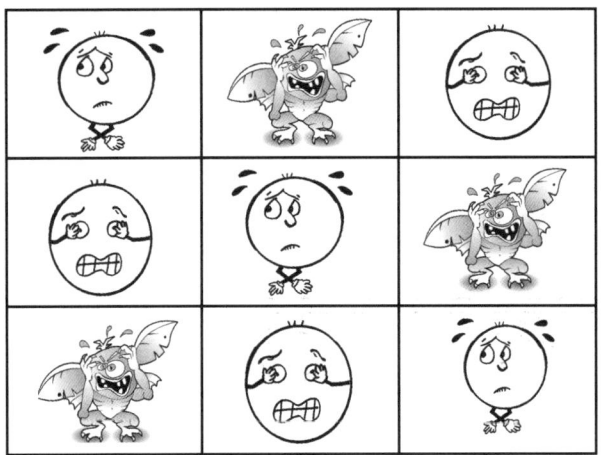

Missing Piece

The missing piece is B.

Starve the Anxiety Gremlin Fill-In Puzzle

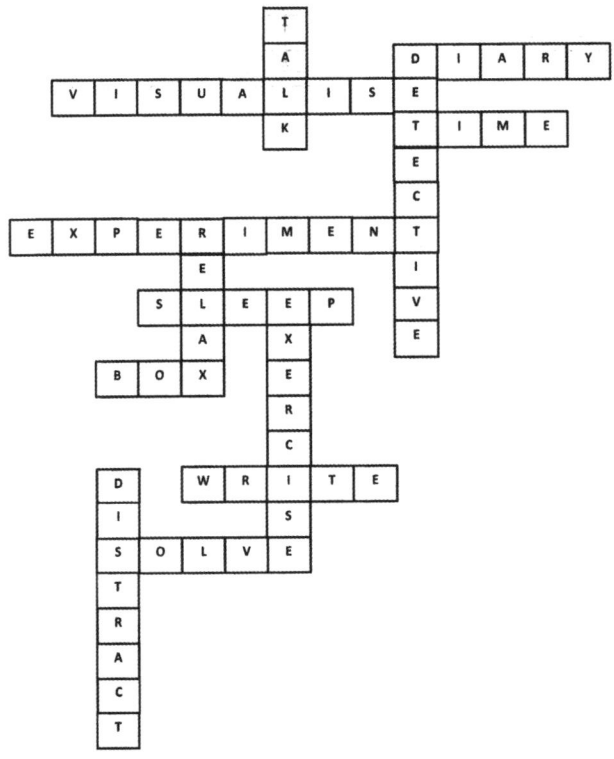

Crack the Code

The message is: STARVE YOUR ANXIETY GREMLIN.
   Here is the completed code grid:

1 = S	2 = R	3 = E
4 = U	5 = N	6 = L
7 = X	△ = A	? = M
⌂ = I	# = Y	+ = G
* = T	☐ = V	@ = O

The Anger Quiz

1. Emotion
2. The odd one out is yawn as it is not a feeling
3. You could have put scared, surprised or sad
4. Feeling
5. True
6. a
7. Flight
8. a. Places   b. People   c. Animals   d. Situations
9. Glasses
10. a and b
11. a, b and c
12. a
13. a
14. a, b and c

The Anxiety Gremlin Fact-File!

The Anxiety **GREMLIN** is a troublesome pest.

The Anxiety Gremlin loves it when you get **ANXIOUS**.

If you think through Anxiety Thinking Glasses, you **FEED** the Anxiety Gremlin.

Anxious physical **FEELINGS** feed the Anxiety Gremlin.

Anxious behaviours that are bad for you feed the **ANXIETY** Gremlin.

The more you **FEED** the Anxiety Gremlin, the bigger he gets.

The **BIGGER** the Anxiety Gremlin gets, the more anxious you get.

The more anxious you get, the more bad effects your **ANXIETY** has on you.

And the **ANXIETY** Gremlin gets even bigger!

But if you think differently and **ACT** differently, you can starve the Anxiety Gremlin.

If you are a **THOUGHT** Detective, you starve the Anxiety Gremlin.

If you are a behaviour **SCIENTIST**, you starve the Anxiety Gremlin.

If you **STARVE** the Anxiety Gremlin, he will get smaller and smaller and you will get less and less anxious!

Information for Parents and Professionals

The Purpose of This Workbook

Starving the Anxiety Gremlin for Children Aged 5–9 provides a cognitive behavioural approach to anxiety management for children aged 5–9 years. The cognitive behavioural approach of this workbook is combined with the approach of a traditional colouring and puzzle book to create an educational yet fun resource. And as children progress through this workbook they can gain fun rewards in the form of **Starving the Anxiety Gremlin Stars** and **Just for Fun Puzzles** as a celebration of their learning and progress.

Starving the Anxiety Gremlin for Children Aged 5–9 is designed for children to work through with the support of a parent or professional, such as a mental health practitioner, teacher, mentor, teaching assistant, social worker or youth worker. The self-help materials included in this workbook are based on the principles of cognitive behavioural therapy (CBT) but do not constitute a session-by-session therapeutic programme. However, the materials contained in this workbook can be used as a resource for therapists working with children.

An evaluation checklist is included in the final chapter of the workbook to enable the child to identify just how much they have learnt and how they have progressed. However, please note that this isn't designed to be used as a clinical diagnostic tool.

Please note that this workbook should not be considered a substitute for professional treatment where required.

What is Cognitive Behavioural Therapy?

CBT is an evidence-based, skills-based, structured form of psychotherapy, which emerged from Beck's Cognitive Therapy (e.g. Beck 1976) and Ellis' Rational-Emotive Therapy (e.g. Ellis 1962), as well as from the work of behaviourists such as Pavlov (e.g. Pavlov 1927) and Skinner (e.g. Skinner 1938) on classical and operant conditioning, respectively. CBT looks at the relationships between our thoughts (cognition), our feelings (emotions) and our actions (behaviours). It is based on the premise that how we interpret experiences and situations has a profound effect on our behaviours and emotions.

CBT focuses on:

- the problems that the client is experiencing in the here and now
- why the problems are occurring
- what strategies the client can use in order to address the problems.

In doing so, the CBT process empowers the client to identify:

- negative, unhealthy and unrealistic patterns of thoughts, perspectives and beliefs
- maladaptive and unhealthy patterns of behaviour
- the links between the problems the client is facing and his or her patterns of thoughts and behaviours
- how to challenge the existing patterns of thoughts and behaviours and implement alternative thoughts and behaviours that are constructive, healthy and realistic in order to address problems, manage emotions and improve wellbeing.

Thus the underlying ethos of CBT is that by addressing unhelpful patterns of thoughts and behaviours, people can change how they feel, how they view themselves, how they interact with others and how they approach life in general – thereby moving from an unhealthy cycle of reactions to a healthy one.

A wide range of empirical studies show CBT to be effective with many mental health disorders, including:

- anxiety (e.g. Cartwright-Hatton *et al.* 2004; James, Soler and Weatherall 2005)

- obsessive compulsive disorder (OCD) (e.g. O'Kearney *et al.* 2006)

- depression (e.g. Klein, Jacobs and Reinecke 2007).

Furthermore, guidelines published by the National Institute for Health and Care Excellence (NICE) recommend the use of CBT for a number of mental health issues, including depression (NICE 2005a) and OCD (NICE 2005b).

EFFECTIVENESS OF CBT FOR CHILDREN AND YOUNG PEOPLE

Although there has been less research conducted on the use of CBT with children and young people than there has been with adults, evidence for its effectiveness is continuing to grow and is being reported in a number of reviews, such as Kazdin and Weisz (1998) and Rapee *et al.* (2000). Randomised clinical trials have shown CBT to be effective with children and young people for the following:

- specific phobias (Silverman *et al.* 1999)

- generalised anxiety disorder (Kendall *et al.* 1997, 2004)

- social phobia (Spence, Donovan and Brechman-Toussaint 2000)

- obsessive compulsive disorder (Barrett, Healy-Farrell and March 2004)

- school refusal (King *et al.* 1998)

- depression (Lewinsohn and Clarke 1999).

References

Barrett, P., Healy-Farrell, L. and March, J.S. (2004) 'Cognitive-behavioural family treatment of childhood obsessive compulsive disorder: a controlled trial.' *Journal of the American Academy of Child and Adolescent Psychiatry 43*, 1, 46–62.
Beck, A.T. (1976) *Cognitive Therapy and Emotional Disorders*. New York: International Universities Press.
Cartwright-Hatton, S., Roberts, C., Chitsabesan, P., Fothergill, C. *et al.* (2004) 'Systematic review of the efficacy of cognitive behaviour therapies for childhood and adolescent anxiety disorders.' *British Journal of Clinical Psychology 43*, 421–436.
Ellis, A. (1962) *Reason and Emotion in Psychotherapy*. New York: Lyle-Stuart.
James, A.A.C.J., Soler, A. and Weatherall, R.R.W. (2005) 'Cognitive behavioural therapy for anxiety disorders in children and adolescents.' *Cochrane Database of Systematic Reviews 2005*, 4, CD004690. DOI: 10.1002/14651858.CD004690.pub2.
Kazdin, A.E. and Weisz, J.R. (1998) 'Identifying and developing empirically supported child and adolescent treatments.' *Journal of Consulting and Clinical Psychology 66*, 19–36.
Kendall, P.C., Flannery-Schroeder, E., Panichelli-Mindel, S.M., Sotham-Gerow, M., Henin, A. and Warman, M. (1997) 'Therapy with youths with anxiety disorders: a second randomized clinical trial.' *Journal of Consulting and Clinical Psychology 18*, 255–270.
Kendall, P.C., Safford, S., Flannery-Schroeder, E. and Webb, A. (2004) 'Child anxiety treatment: outcomes in adolescence and impact on substance abuse and depression at 7.4 year follow-up.' *Journal of Consulting and Clinical Psychology 72*, 276–287.
King, N.J., Molloy, G.N., Heyme, D., Murphy, G.C. and Ollendick, T. (1998) 'Emotive imagery treatment for childhood phobias: a credible and empirically validated intervention?' *Behavioural and Cognitive Psychotherapy 26*, 103–113.
Klein, J.B., Jacobs, R.H. and Reinecke, M.A. (2007) 'A meta-analysis of CBT in adolescents with depression.' *Journal of the American Academy of Child and Adolescent Psychiatry 46*, 1403–1413.
Lewinsohn, P.M. and Clarke, G.N. (1999) 'Psychosocial treatments for adolescent depression.' *Clinical Psychology Review 19*, 329–42.
National Institute for Health and Care Excellence (NICE) (2005a) 'Depression in children and young people: identification and management in primary, community and secondary care.' *Clinical Guideline* 28. Available at www.nice.org.uk/guidance/CG28, accessed on 2 May 2014.
National Institute for Health and Care Excellence (NICE) (2005b) 'Obsessive compulsive disorder: core interventions in the treatment of obsessive compulsive disorder and body dysmorphic disorder.' *Clinical Guideline* 31. Available at www.nice.org.uk/nicemedia/pdf/CG031niceguideline.pdf, accessed on 2 May 2014.
O'Kearney, R.T., Anstey, K., von Sanden, C. and Hunt, A. (2006) 'Behavioural and cognitive behavioural therapy for obsessive compulsive disorder in children and adolescents.' *Cochrane Database of Systematic Reviews 2006*, 4, CD004856. DOI: 10.1002/14651858.CD004856.pub2.
Pavlov, I.P. (1927) *Conditioned Reflexes: An Investigation of the Physiological Activity of the Cerebral Cortex*. Translated and edited by G. V. Anrep. London: Oxford University Press.
Rapee, R.M., Wignall, A., Hudson, J.L. and Schniering, C.A. (2000) *Treating Anxious Children and Adolescents: An Evidence-Based Approach*. Oakland, CA: New Harbinger Publications.
Silverman, W.K., Kurtines, W.M., Ginsburg, G.S., Weems, C.F., Rabian, B. and Setafini, L.T. (1999) 'Contingency management, self-control and education support in the treatment of childhood phobic disorders: a randomized clinical trial.' *Journal of Consulting and Clinical Psychology 67*, 675–687.
Skinner, B.F. (1938) *The Behavior of Organisms*. New York: Appleton-Century-Crofts.
Spence, S., Donovan, C. and Brechman-Toussaint, M. (2000) 'The treatment of childhood social phobia: the effectiveness of a social skills training-based cognitive behavioural intervention with and without parental involvement.' *Journal of Child Psychology and Psychiatry 41*, 713–726.